Studies in Laboratory Phonology

In this series:

5. Bergmann, Pia. Morphologisch komplexe Wörter im Deutschen: Prosodische Struktur und phonetische Realisierung.
6. Feldhausen, Ingo, Jan Fliessbach & Maria del Mar Vanrell (eds.). Methods in prosody: A Romance language perspective.
7. Tilsen, Sam. Syntax with oscillators and energy levels.
8. Ben Hedia, Sonia. Gemination and degemination in English affixation: Investigating the interplay between morphology, phonology and phonetics.
9. Easterday, Shelece. Highly complex syllable structure: A typological and diachronic study.
10. Roessig, Simon. Categoriality and continuity in prosodic prominence.
11. Schmitz, Dominic. Production, perception, and comprehension of subphonemic detail: Word-Final /s/ in English.
12. Schubö, Fabian, Sabine Zerbian, Sandra Hanne & Isabell Wartenburger (eds.). Prosodic boundary phenomena.
13. Albert, Aviad. A model of sonority based on pitch intelligibility.
14. Wehrle, Simon. Conversation and intonation in autism: A multi-dimensional analysis.

ISSN: 2363-5576

Conversation and intonation in autism

A multi-dimensional analysis

Simon Wehrle

language
science
press

Simon Wehrle. 2023. *Conversation and intonation in autism: A multi-dimensional analysis* (Studies in Laboratory Phonology 14). Berlin: Language Science Press.

This title can be downloaded at:
http://langsci-press.org/catalog/book/404

The work presented in this book is based on the author's doctoral dissertation, which was accepted by the Faculty of Arts and Humanities at the University of Cologne in 2021.
ISBN: 978-3-96110-426-0 (Digital)
978-3-98554-084-6 (Hardcover)

ISSN: 2363-5576
DOI: 10.5281/zenodo.10069004
Source code available from www.github.com/langsci/404
Errata: paperhive.org/documents/remote?type=langsci&id=404

Cover and concept of design: Ulrike Harbort
Typesetting: Simon Wehrle
Fonts: Libertinus, Arimo, DejaVu Sans Mono
Typesetting software: XƎLaTeX

Language Science Press
xHain
Grünberger Str. 16
10243 Berlin, Germany
http://langsci-press.org

Storage and cataloguing done by FU Berlin

Freie Universität Berlin

Contents

Acknowledgments

This book is a revised and improved version of the doctoral dissertation I submitted in October 2021. The original acknowledgments are reprinted below with minor (though in at least one case momentous) updates.

This work would quite simply and quite literally not have been possible without the doctoral scholarship I have had the privilege to receive. I would therefore like to thank the *Studienstiftung des deutschen Volkes* (German Academic Scholarship Foundation) for their very generous and patient support, even in the face of more or less foreseeable vagaries such as parenthood and a global pandemic. I am also very grateful to the SFB 1252 at the University of Cologne. My membership in this collaborative research centre has benefitted me in a number of very different but equally important ways.

Massive thanks also to my doctoral supervisors, Martine Grice and Kai Vogeley. Martine has supported and inspired me since I first cautiously stepped into the Cologne phonetics lab and has been an extraordinarily approachable, helpful and insightful supervisor and human being. I am very grateful to Kai for lending some of his vast expertise to my project and for always being open-minded and encouraging in discussions of my research. Big thanks to Stefan Baumann for agreeing to be my third examiner, for being a great colleague and for closing the circle from leading the very first MA seminar I attended to the completion of this book.

I can't give enough thanks to Franceso Cangemi, my "shadow supervisor" and, dare I say it, mentor (sorry for making you sound old). Francesco has had a hand in the germination of most valuable ideas expressed in this book. More importantly, I am grateful for the many, many deep, fun, silly, serious, musical, scientific and all-of-the-above hours we shared. Big thanks, too, to the third Swiss Sister, Aviad Albert, for sharing musical adventures and fun discussions with me, but also for massively helping me with some of the more technical aspects of this book in particular.

Thanks to many other Cologne people past and current, all with undue brevity: Martina Krüger for getting me started on the autism data, Kieu-Phuong Glaser (Ha) for getting me into backchannels, and Malin Spaniol for brilliantly leading the way into the next phase of research and for generally being a great person to be around. To Alicia Janz, Harriet Hanekamp, Matthias Gauser and Anika Müller for their invaluable help with data, annotation, breakfasts, dog-sitting and more. Thanks to Christine Röhr for being an exemplary and open-minded gatekeeper and colleague. To Simona Sbranna and Eduardo Möking for keeping me in touch with and excited about the L2 world. Thanks to Juliane Zimmermann for lots of insightful and fun discussions; thanks also to her psychiatry colleagues Valeria Lucarini, Carola Bloch, Mathis Jording and David Vogel.

Outside my immediate surroundings, I want to first give special thanks to the dynamic duo of Bodo Winter and Timo Roettger. Bodo might not know this, but he's been a great "enabler" in the best sense for me through the years, having at various points given me encouragement and advice that has often proved invaluable in hindsight. He has also greatly contributed to the methodological fine-tuning of the backchannel and filled pause analysis and his sharp mind rarely fails to deliver some valuable insight even during the shortest of exchanges. Timo has been a great collaborator in the past and is a role model for his dedication to high-quality open science as well as to most other things that are not broken in academia. Together, Bodo and Timo have opened my eyes many years ago to the importance of statistical analysis, while also fuelling my existing passion for clear and beautiful data visualisation. Finally, they have both contributed to my shift from the NHST framework I never liked or subscribed to in the first place to embracing the Bayesian mindset (all via the strange no man's land of pure description and exploration which I am stubbornly keeping one foot in).

I would like to thank Nigel Ward for the collaboration on prosodic constructions and his many influential written works – to be continued. Many other people have been kind enough to share their thoughts on this project with me and provided valuable feedback, including Mark Dingemanse, Riccardo Fusaroli, Elina Savino, Francisco Torreira, Jason Bishop, Gemma Williams, Loulou Kosmala, Mattias Heldner, Katharina Zahner-Ritter, Bob Ladd and Bettina Braun. Special thanks to Olcay Türk, Sasha Calhoun and Paul Warren for hosting me in Wellington.

Back in Cologne, many people have contributed to making the phonetics lab a special place over the years, in every sense and at various points. In no particular order and under no illusions of completeness, thank you to: Theo Klinker, Anna Bruggeman, Lena Pagel, Tabea Thies, Maria Lialiou, Janne Lorenzen, Jane Mertens, Christine Riek, Simon Roessig, Caterina Ventura, Esther Weitz, Mark Ellison, Anne Hermes, Doris Mücke, Constantijn Kaland, Katinka Wüllner, Noemi Furlani, Chem Vatho, Janina Kalbertodt, Mathias Stöber, Georg Sachse, Drenushë Valera-Kurteshi and Jessica di Napoli. Special thanks to the participants of the FORAUS discussion forum for autistic adults, who generously shared their lived experiences and thereby deeply informed my interpretation of the experimental results and analyses.

Even closer to home, I am very grateful to my parents for their unwavering support, no matter how comprehensible or sensible my path may have seemed at times. Danke für alles. Thanks also to Betti and Chrissi for being excellent sisters. Flip gets a pat for outstanding moral support and swampy breath and for a brief but stellar stint as the lab lap dog.

Finally, ultimately, to Rachel, Wilbur and Ida. Wilbur, who blew my mind upon arrival and has been helping me to reassemble it in a better form ever since. You continue to inspire, challenge and delight me every day. And Ida, who has been pushing the envelope in her own delightful way, at once squishable and regal. Above it all, Rachel: you deserve endless credit for having been entirely patient and gracious throughout this long and sometimes arduous process and far beyond it. It would take me another 218 pages to produce the mere outline of a rough sketch of everything you mean to me and of how grateful I am to you. As I imagine this would be deemed inappropriate here, I will restrict myself to saying: thank you so much, for everything, always.

1 General introduction

The overall aim in this book is to analyse the conversation strategies and intonation styles of German adults with and without a diagnosis of autism spectrum disorder (ASD) in order to arrive at a better characterisation of communicative behaviour in ASD. I provide an in-depth, multi-dimensional analysis focussing on the dimensions of intonation style, turn-taking, backchannels, filled pauses and silent pauses (along other parameters). Speakers engaged in semi-structured spontaneous conversation were recorded in two groups of disposition-matched speaker pairs (i.e. interlocutors either both did or did not have a diagnosis of ASD).

In this first chapter, I will give a very brief overview of ASD in general and communication in ASD in particular before providing an outline of the book and anticipating some of the most important findings.

1.1 The autism spectrum: Overview and terminology

The leading diagnostic manuals DSM-5 and ICD-11 describe autism spectrum disorder as a neurodevelopmental disorder that is characterised by "deficits in social interaction and communication" as well as "repetitive, restricted behaviours and interests" (American Psychiatric Association 2013, World Health Organization 2022). The estimated prevalence of ASD is around 1% (Christensen et al. 2018, Elsabbagh et al. 2012).[1]

In the most recent classifications, the previously used subgroups of *Asperger syndrome* and *high-functioning autism* have been subsumed under the single category of autism spectrum disorder. Asperger syndrome as defined in ICD-10 (F84.5) refers to individuals with an IQ of over 70 and no delays in language acquisition and cognitive development. High-functioning autism is a term that is not actually included in either the DSM-5 or the ICD-10, but has commonly been used to refer to autistic individuals with an average or above-average IQ who, in

[1]Please note that while I explicitly do not follow a deficit-based view of autism in this work, I may make reference to such views in referring to the current diagnostic criteria and to descriptions in the previous literature.

contrast to individuals with Asperger syndrome, did experience a delay in language acquisition (see Krüger 2018: Chapter 4). As most research suggests that a reliable differentiation between autism spectrum disorder and the proposed subcategories of high-functioning autism and Asperger syndrome is indeed not possible (Frazier et al. 2012, Lord et al. 2012), I will be referring only to the overarching category of ASD throughout this book (even though the ICD-10 diagnosis F84.5 (Asperger syndrome) was applied at the time of diagnosis for all autistic participants in the corpus under study).

Differences in communicative behaviour are a core characteristic of ASD, and the one that is most relevant to the work presented in this book. Although, typically for ASD, individual differences abound, some overarching trends in the use of gaze, gesture and language in ASD have been identified. Very broadly speaking, these include more differences in the social, rather than functional aspects of language (see Krüger 2018), characteristic patterns in both the production and perception of prosody (e.g. McCann & Peppé 2003, Paul et al. 2005, Grice et al. 2023) and a more literal (rather than figurative) use and understanding of language (e.g. Happé 1995).

It is important to note that many of these findings have been made predominantly or exclusively on the basis of data from children and adolescents (see Krüger 2018, Grice et al. 2023). As we know 1) that language skills often improve throughout early life in ASD (Gernsbacher et al. 2016) and 2) that there is a general lack of research into communication by autistic adults, it is not always clear to what extent such findings apply to adults with ASD (including the speakers in the corpus analysed here).

I will provide detailed accounts of the aspects of communication in ASD that are most relevant to the findings presented in this book in the following chapters, along with the relevant experimental results.

Regarding terminology, I refer to e.g. *autistic individuals* or people *on the autism spectrum* rather than to *individuals with ASD* in this book. In other words, I have chosen to use identity-first rather than person-first language. Although there have increasingly been calls for an exclusive use of identity-first language (*autistic person*) in recent years, there is no complete consensus on the matter (Botha et al. 2021, Bottema-Beutel et al. 2021, Dunn & Andrews 2015, Gernsbacher 2017, Vivanti 2020, Tepest 2021). I acknowledge this ambiguity and hope that those who prefer the use of person-first language can see past these matters of terminology and still benefit from the insights put forward in this book.

On a similar note, it is worth pointing out that I will draw on research into bilingual or second-language communication as a point of comparison with communication in ASD in some parts of this book. This is done mainly due to a considerable, or in some cases even complete, lack of previous research on relevant aspects of communication in ASD. The comparison with second-language speech strikes me as fruitful and well-motivated in many respects, but I am of course acutely aware of the crucial differences between non-native speakers and autistic persons in terms of developmental trajectories and neurobiology (among others). It is simply my hope that this comparison can elucidate some phenotypical similarities between the two groups and that it may even be possible to transfer some of the knowledge and resources from the well-established research fields of bilingual and cross-cultural communication to the benefit of research on autistic and cross-neurotype communication.

Having established these basic concepts and some important terminological choices, I will proceed to give an overview of the data and methods used in Chapter 2 following the outline of the remaining parts of this book presented in the next section.

1.2 Synopsis: Dimensions of conversation and intonation in ASD

In Chapter 3, *intonation style* is investigated. Since the very beginnings of research into ASD, there have been contradicting descriptions of speech in ASD as being either particularly melodic or particularly monotonous. A novel methodology, designed to avoid shortcomings of previous acoustic analyses, was used to reliably quantify intonation styles in ASD. It is shown that ASD speakers in the corpus under study tended to produce a more melodic intonation style than non-autistic control (CTR) speakers, while none produced a more monotonous intonation style. It is further shown that the proposed method for quantifying intonation styles is at least equivalent to previous efforts relying on parameters such as pitch range and span and superior to accounts relying solely on mean fundamental frequency.

Chapter 4 is dedicated to an analysis of *turn-taking*. The organisation of who speaks when in conversation is perhaps the most fundamental aspect of human communication. Previous research on a wide variety of speakers has revealed a seemingly universal preference for between-speaker transitions consisting of very short silent gaps. Research on turn-taking in ASD is very limited to date, and no studies have investigated dialogues between autistic adults. It is shown that turn-timing was very similar in the CTR and the ASD group overall, but also that autistic dyads produced unusually long silent gaps in the early stages of dialogue. Further evidence reveals that ASD dyads reacted differently to unexpected events in conversation, that speaking times were less balanced within ASD dyads, and that the prosodic realisation of turn ends and beginnings seems to be identical across groups.

A number of related phenomena are described in Chapter 5, all of which play particularly important roles in dialogue management. First, it is shown in §5.3 that *backchannels* (listener signals such as *mmhm* or *okay*), which in the context of ASD have not been investigated in any detail to date, were produced in unusual ways by ASD dyads. Compared to the CTR group, the ASD group produced a lower rate of backchannels (especially in the early stages of dialogue), used a less diverse range of different backchannel types and showed a less complex mapping of different intonation contours to different backchannel types. Second, it is shown in §5.4 that *filled pauses* (hesitation signals such as *uhm*), contrary to most previous results, did not differ between groups in rate or choice of filled pause type (*uh* or *uhm*). For prosodic realisation (which had not been investigated in previous studies), it was found that ASD dyads produced fewer filled pauses with the prototypical level intonation. Third, it is shown in §5.5 and §5.6 that ASD dyads produced more long *silent pauses* and a lower rate of *laughter*.

Chapter 6 provides the *conclusion* of the book, in which I first propose a summary analysis. This provides an in-depth description of the communicative behaviour of each ASD dyad, while also highlighting differences and similarities across autistic dyads compared to the CTR group, along all dimensions of conversation and intonation investigated. After summarising the most important findings, emphasising the important role of individual- and dyad-specific variability and discussing which behaviours seem to be most characteristic of communication in ASD, I end by reflecting on the external validity of the results presented and on future avenues of investigation.

2 Data and methods

In the following, I will provide details on the subjects that participated in this study as well as on experimental methods and materials. Further, I will present the chosen approach of combining in-depth exploratory analysis with Bayesian modelling.

2.1 Participants

For the corpus used throughout this book, 28 monolingual native speakers of German (14 ASD, 14 CTR) were recorded performing Map Tasks (see §2.2) in homogeneous, disposition-matched dyads (7 ASD–ASD, 7 CTR–CTR). Participants from the ASD group had all been diagnosed with Asperger syndrome (ICD-10: F84.5) and were recruited in the Autism Outpatient Clinic at the Department of Psychiatry, University of Cologne (Germany). As part of a systematic assessment implemented in the clinic, diagnoses were made independently by two different specialised clinicians corresponding to ICD-10 criteria and supplemented by an extensive neuropsychological assessment.

Subjects from the ASD group were first recorded and described by Krüger (2018) and Krüger et al. (2018) (performing different tasks). Participants from the control group were recruited from the general population specifically for this study. All subjects were paid 10 EUR for participation. It was ascertained that participants had not been acquainted with each other before the start of the experiment (although some participants in the ASD group may have crossed paths in the context of the autism outpatient clinic).

Disposition-matched dyads (ASD–ASD; CTR–CTR) rather than mixed dyads (ASD–CTR) were recorded for two main reasons. First, there is a dramatic lack of research on communication in ASD based on data from matched rather than mixed dyads. Second, investigating the behaviour of disposition-matched dyads seems to us the most promising way to gain insights into what we might justifiably call autistic communication. Analysing the behaviour of mixed dyads makes it very difficult to see beyond patterns arising from the divergent behaviour of individuals with different cognitive styles. While such insights are of great value in principle, they cannot be interpreted accurately unless we first have a clear picture of what characterises communication in disposition-matched autistic dyads (see e.g. §4.5.3 for further discussion). Indeed, recent research suggests that many social difficulties experienced by people on the autism spectrum might, in fact, be due to neurotype mismatches (arising in interactions with non-autistic people) rather than any inherent cognitive "deficits" or "impairments" (Crompton et al. 2020, Morrison et al. 2020, Rifai et al. 2022). This perspective reflects a growing (and perhaps overdue) broader awareness that analyses of interaction, rather than of isolated minds, should be at the core of cognitive science, linguistics and related disciplines (Dingemanse et al. 2023).

All participants completed the German version of the Autism-Spectrum Quotient (AQ) questionnaire, an instrument developed by Baron-Cohen et al. (2001) to measure autistic traits in adults with "normal" intelligence. AQ scores range from 0 to 50, with higher scores indicating more autistic traits. An AQ score of 32 or above is commonly interpreted as a clinical threshold for ASD (Ashwood et al. 2016, Baron-Cohen et al. 2001).

All participants also completed the 'Wortschatztest WST' (Schmidt & Metzler 1992), a standardised, receptive German vocabulary test that exhibits a high correlation not only with verbal intelligence, but also with general intelligence (Satzger et al. 2002).

Although participants from the CTR group were matched as closely as possible to the ASD group for age, verbal IQ and gender, some minor differences remained.

Participants from the ASD group were on average slightly older (mean = 44; range: 31–55) than participants from the CTR group (mean = 37; range: 29–54). However, there was extensive overlap between groups and, moreover, there is no a priori reason to assume that such a relatively small difference in this particular age range would act as a confound in group comparisons. Bayesian modelling confirmed the age difference between groups as a robust effect (with the ASD group as the reference level: mean δ = -7.12; 95% CI [-11.06, -3.22]; posterior probability $P(\delta > 0) = 1$). More information on the use of Bayesian modelling in this book can be found in §2.3; details on the specific models used here are found in the accompanying scripts and files (see the *Open Science Framework (OSF)* repository at https://osf.io/6vynj/).

Further, the ASD group had a slightly higher average verbal IQ score (mean = 118; range: 101–143) than the CTR group (mean = 106; range: 99–118). Again, there was considerable overlap between groups. There is no reason to assume that this difference should have a meaningful impact on results. Bayesian modelling confirmed the difference in verbal IQ as a robust effect (with the ASD group as the reference level: mean δ = -12.31; 95% CI [-18.7, -5.67]; posterior probability $P(\delta > 0) = 1$).

The gender ratio was similar, but not identical across groups. The ASD group contained 4 females and 10 males, whereas the CTR group contained 3 females and 11 males. This entails that dialogues took place in the ASD group between 1 all-female dyad, 2 mixed dyads and 4 all-male dyads, but in the CTR group between 3 mixed dyads and 4 all-male dyads (i.e. no all-female dyad). Bayesian modelling confirms that these small differences between groups did not, however, have any notable effects on results in any of the areas under investigation. Details can be found in the relevant chapters.

Most importantly, there was a clear difference in AQ scores between groups, with a far higher average score in the ASD group (mean = 41.9; range = 35–46) than in the CTR group (mean = 16.1; range: 11–26) and no overlap at all between subjects from both groups. All subjects in the ASD group scored above the suggested threshold of 32 points and all subjects in the CTR group scored below the same threshold. Bayesian modelling provides unambiguous evidence for the group difference in AQ scores (with the ASD group as the reference level: mean δ = -25.83; 95% CI [-29.03, -22.67]; posterior probability $P(\delta > 0) = 1$).

Table 2.1 shows summary statistics for gender, age, verbal IQ and AQ.

Table 2.1: Subject information by group. SD = Standard deviation.

	Gender (n)		Age		Verbal IQ		AQ	
	female	male	Mean	SD	Mean	SD	Mean	SD
ASD	4	10	43.6	6.7	118.1	12.0	41.9	3.1
CTR	3	11	36.5	7.6	105.8	5.8	16.1	4.5

All aspects of the study were approved by the local ethics committee of the Medical Faculty at the University of Cologne and were performed in accordance with the ethical standards laid down in the 1964 Declaration of Helsinki and its later amendments. All participants gave their written informed consent prior to participating in the experiment.

2.2 Materials and procedure

Map Tasks were used to elicit semi-spontaneous speech. The Map Task paradigm was introduced by Anderson et al. (1984) and has widely been used in speech research for over 30 years (for an influential article describing a corpus of Map Task speech see Anderson et al. 1991).

The Map Task paradigm was chosen for the current investigation as it provides us with predominantly spontaneous speech data that can, however, still be controlled along a number of key parameters, such as lexical items (via the names of landmarks on a map) and communicative obstacles (such as the introduction of mismatching landmarks between maps; see below for more detail). While the elicited dialogues are not fully free or spontaneous, the Map Task was determined to be a good choice in the context of comparing autistic and non-autistic dyads, since the constraints involved in the task serve to reduce a potentially particularly high degree of variability across the autism spectrum in terms of social motivation, interest in a given topic, and the adherence to social conventions.

Participants were recorded in pairs (dyads). After filling in a number of forms and the questionnaires listed in §2.1, participants received written instructions for the task and entered a recording booth. Each participant was presented with a simple map containing nine landmark items in the form of small pictures (materials adapted from Grice & Savino 2003). Only one of the two participants (the instruction giver) had a route printed on their map. The experimental task was for the instruction follower to transfer this route to their own map by exchanging information with the instruction giver.

During this entire process, an opaque screen was placed between participants, meaning they could not establish visual contact and had to solve the task by means of verbal communication alone. The roles of instruction giver and instruction follower were assigned randomly. Upon completion of the first task, the participants received a new set of maps and their roles were switched. The task ended once the second Map Task was completed.

As participants were naive to the purpose of the study, they did not know (initially) that their maps differed in some crucial regards. In each map, some landmarks were either missing, duplicated and/or replaced with a different landmark compared to the interlocutor's map. This was the case for two landmarks per map in the experiment. Those items that differed between maps will hereafter be called Mismatches (or mismatching landmarks); items that were the same on both maps will be called Matches (or matching landmarks).

During annotation, the portion of dialogue in which the first Mismatch was discussed by participants was marked and this was used to divide all dialogues up into three epochs, i.e., before detection, during discussion, and after resolution of the first Mismatch. This was expanded to a continuous analysis or reduced to a binary distinction as appropriate. Further details can be found in the discussion of relevant findings in the following chapters (e.g. §3.4.4, §4.4.1.3 and §5.3.2.1).

An example of maps used in this study is shown in Figure 2.1, with Mismatches highlighted using red circles. All dyads received the same two pairs of maps.

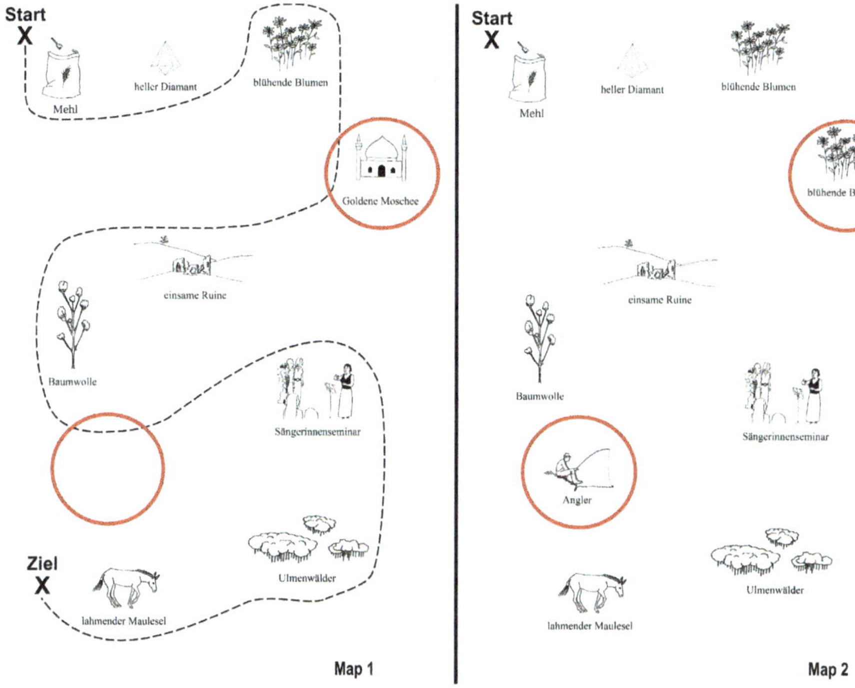

Figure 2.1: One pair of maps used in the study. The instruction giver's map, with a route leading from 'Start' (top left) to 'Ziel' (finish; bottom left), is in the left panel. Mismatches between maps are highlighted with red circles.

Map Task conversations were recorded in a sound-proof booth at the Department of Phonetics, University of Cologne. Two head-mounted microphones (AKG C420L) connected through an audio-interface (PreSonus AudioBox 22VSL) to a PC running Adobe Audition were used. The sample rate was 44100 Hz (16 bit). Recordings were transcribed orthographically and divided into inter-pausal units (IPUs) with a minimum pause length of 200 ms (De Jong & Bosker 2013, Goldman-Eisler 1968, Cho & Hirst 2006).

Only recorded dialogue from the start to the end of each task was included in all analyses in order to achieve a greater degree of comparability regarding conversational context and content. The total duration of all edited dialogues was 4 hours and 44 minutes. The mean dialogue duration was 20 minutes and 19 seconds (SD = 12'32"; for detailed information and analysis see §4.4.4.2). Note that far less time would have been necessary to simply complete the task at hand for most dyads. A qualitative analysis confirmed that most participants engaged in a very free mode of conversation, rather than strictly working through the two Map Tasks – although there were some intriguing group differences in this regard, with ASD dyads seeming to lean more towards a task-oriented style of conversation (see results in the following chapters for more details).

Figure 2.2 shows an example excerpt of Map Task dialogue from one of the ASD dyads, transcribed following GAT conventions (see Couper-Kuhlen & Barth-Weingarten 2011). Phenomena that are of particular interest for the following analyses are highlighted in bold: two backchannels, one filled pause and two turn transitions (one following the introduction of a matching landmark – 'heller Diamant' (bright diamond), line 15/16 – and one following the introduction of a mismatching landmark – 'goldene Moschee' (golden mosque), line 21/22). Note that the turn transitions highlighted here are considerably longer than average transitions between turns (cf. Chapter 4).

2.3 Principles of analysis

This section will give details on the general principles and methods of analysis used throughout this book. Details applicable to specific measurements can be found in the relevant subchapters.

2.3.1 The importance of individual specificity

One of the guiding principles in this work is a commitment to in-depth analyses appropriately accounting for inter-individual variability and dyad-specific behaviour (cf. Bruggeman et al. 2017, Cangemi et al. 2016, 2015). The importance of considering scientific data at the level of the individual (and the dyad) is not limited to this study, nor to the fields of linguistics and psychology. It is, however, made all the more critical when we aim to describe and understand the behaviour of a group of speakers as intrinsically heterogeneous as any group composed of individuals diagnosed with ASD. This point is taken up again throughout the book (see in particular §6.1.2 and §6.2.1).

A large number of findings have shown evidence for a particularly high degree of heterogeneity in groups of individuals diagnosed with ASD (e.g. Wozniak et al. 2017). This heterogeneity is at the very core of what is by definition a spectrum disorder with a continuous distribution of features and properties (American Psychiatric Association 2013). One underlying reason for this heterogeneity

```
13      S1:     (-) okay   du    gehst unter dem mehl durch
                    okay   you    go  under the flour through
                     'okay you pass below the flour'

14      S2:     j  ja                 → Backchannel
                y  yes

15      S1:     °h in richtung  heller diamant
                   in direction bright diamond
                'towards the bright diamond'

→ 1738 ms gap (Match)

16      S2:     °hhh okay             → Backchannel

17      S1:     dann gehst du o:bm     über die blu blühenden  blumen und zwar
wirklich über   die blumen
                then  go  you above   over the flo-blossoming flowers and indeed
really   above  the flowers
                'then you go above the blossoming flowers, really above the flowers'

18              nicht  über  die (.) äh über  die buchstaben          → Filled Pause
                not    above the     uh above the letters
                'not above the writing'

19      S2:     achso    über  die blühenden  blumen  ja
                oh right above the blossoming flowers yes
                'I see, above the blossoming flowers, yes'

20      S1:     oben drüber [dann ge]hst du runter °hh [gehst] an der goldenen moschee
vorbei
                up    above [then  go]  you down       [go]   at the golden     mosque
past
                'above it, then you go down, you go past the golden mosque'

21      S2:                 [ja]                  [runter]
                            [yes]                  [down]

→ 971 ms gap (Mismatch)

22              °hhh goldene moschee
                     golden  mosque

23      S1:     (-) ja °hhh du  gehst [weiter] runter an der einsamen
                   yes      you go   [further] down   at the  lonely
                'yes you go further down, past the lonely'

24      S2:                               [hmm]

25              ich hab aber hier keine goldene moschee
                i   have but here no     golden  mosque
                'but I don't have a golden mosque here'

26      S1:     (-) du  hast keine goldene moschee
                    you have no    golden  mosque

27      S2:     nein
                no

28      S1:     °hh dann hast du   eine andere    landkarte
                    then have you  a    different map
                'then you've got a different map'
```

Figure 2.2: Example excerpt of a GAT transcription, with backchannels, filled pauses, and turn transitions following newly introduced landmarks highlighted in bold.

is the fact that autistic people can be expected to adapt less than their non-autistic peers to certain specific and shifting cultural and linguistic conventions at any one point in time. We cannot always disentangle whether this might be due to a lack of interest or ability in specific cases, but the effect is that idiosyncratic aspects of speech and communication in ASD are likely to be magnified when held up to the current conventions of the non-autistic mainstream.

While individual-specific analysis can be seen an asset for any study of human behaviour and is particularly relevant for investigations into ASD, it becomes nothing less than a necessity when we are additionally faced with relatively small sample sizes, as has been the case in the vast majority of studies on communication in ASD. In this area of research, it is very unlikely that any individual study will reach the minimum sample size of 100 participants that has recently been claimed to be a requirement for achieving adequate statistical power (within conventional statistical frameworks) (Brysbaert 2020). While this claim is based on models from the related field of bilingualism research, it can easily be applied to autism research as well.

The problem is in fact only more acute in the case of ASD. There are dramatically fewer autistic people in the world (around 1% of the general population) than there are bilinguals (billions). In this light, openly and deliberately conducting exploratory studies using descriptive analyses, ideally supported by Bayesian methods of statistical inference, seems to me the only reasonable and responsible course of action (Grieve 2021, Tukey 1980, Vasishth, Mertzen, et al. 2018, Yarkoni 2022). Certainly, a single-minded pursuit of sufficiently diminutive p-values in the conventional framework of null-hypothesis significance testing cannot be the solution to this particular problem. The next section spells out some of the issues surrounding the conventional use of frequentist statistical inference and how suggestions for how they may be overcome through a combination of openly exploratory analyses and Bayesian modelling.

2.3.2 In-depth exploration with Bayesian foundations

In reporting experimental results, I emphasise a fully transparent and visually rich descriptive analysis combined with applications of Bayesian modelling and inference. I aim to provide a comprehensive understanding of results first through detailed description and the extensive use of data visualisation (Anscombe 1973, Matejka & Fitzmaurice 2017). Bayesian inference is used in the spirit of complementing, not superseding the descriptive, exploratory analysis that I consider to be at the heart of this work. Therefore, not all details of Bayesian modelling are reported for all analyses, but all information can be found in the accompanying *OSF* repository (see below).

Given the severe lack of reliable previous research and relevant pilot data concerning the phenomena of interest in this book, the analyses presented are necessarily exploratory rather than confirmatory in nature. In this situation, formally testing previously formulated hypotheses using frequentist methods would inherently involve an increased risk of disseminating spurious results based on Type I errors.

Although frequentist inference is still the dominant approach to statistical analysis across different scientific fields, the use of this framework, along with a predominant focus on statistical significance and confirmatory rather than exploratory studies, is associated with a number of grave and wide-ranging issues. These are often summarised under the term *questionable research practices* and go far beyond the specifics of this book. The reader is referred to the growing literature that has been persuasively describing this set of problems as well as the underlying causes and suggestions for possible solutions (e.g. Smaldino & McElreath 2016, Coretta et al. 2023, Amrhein et al. 2019, Bishop 2019, Head et al. 2015, John et al. 2012, Roettger et al. 2019, Roettger 2019).

While Bayesian inference does not in itself prevent the use of such questionable practices, it is an ideal alternative for two main reasons. First, given the limited sample size of the study at hand as well as the lack of previous research on the topic, I have deemed presenting the current results and analyses as exploratory, rather than confirmatory, as the only justifiable option (as discussed in the preceding section). I believe that it would be greatly advantageous for more research in linguistics and related fields to take this approach, rather than presenting as confirmatory work that truly is not (Kerr 1998, Murphy & Aguinis 2019). Bayesian inference is particularly well suited to studies with a limited sample size, as this limitation can be directly reflected in the model output (e.g. in the form of larger credible intervals and a lower posterior probability).

Bayesian inference gives outcomes based on the data at hand, the chosen model and the specified prior assumptions. Compared to frequentist inference, it is therefore, when properly applied, more conservative, but also more robust and transparent in ways that frequentist approaches never are and indeed cannot be, partly because they implicitly treat any given experiment as one in an infinite series of equivalent experiments (Gelman et al. 2020, Lemoine 2019, McElreath 2020, Winter & Bürkner 2021).

Second, Bayesian inference is rapidly increasing in popularity in linguistics and many other fields. This is due in part to practical reasons. Statistical software, tutorials and packages such as the ones used in this book (detailed in the following paragraph) have made the application of Bayesian multilevel modelling increasingly straightforward and at the same time considerably more robust and flexible than the frequentist alternatives (Eager & Roy 2017). Additionally, Bayesian methods seem to be much more closely aligned with common human intuitions and ways of reasoning about the interpretation of statistical tests in general and the notion of significance in particular (Dienes 2011, McShane & Gal 2017, Winter & Bürkner 2021).

I used Bayesian multilevel linear models implemented in the modelling language *Stan* (Carpenter et al. 2017) via the package *brms* for the statistical computing language *R*, which was used in the software *RStudio* (Bürkner 2017, R Core Team 2022, RStudio Team 2021).

Analysis and presentation of Bayesian modelling broadly follows the example of Franke & Roettger (2019), but is also informed by a number of other tutorials (McElreath 2020, Vasishth, Nicenboim, et al. 2018, Winter & Bürkner 2021).

Expected values ($\hat{\beta}$) under the posterior distribution and their 95% credible intervals (CIs) are reported, along with the posterior probability that a difference δ is greater than zero. In essence, a 95% CI represents the range within which an effect is expected to fall with a probability of 95%. Analyses in this book loosely follow the guideline that, if a hypothesis states that $\delta > 0$, there is (strong) support for this hypothesis if zero is (by a reasonably clear margin) not included in the 95% CI of δ and the posterior $P(\delta > 0)$ is close to one (cf. Franke & Roettger 2019). I use this guideline primarily to ensure comparability with conventional null-hypothesis significance testing and reporting practices, but consider 95% credible intervals in and of themselves as the most relevant outcome of Bayesian modelling.

Regularising weakly informative priors were used for all models (Lemoine 2019). Unless otherwise specified, four sampling chains ran for 4000 iterations with a warm-up period of 2000 iterations for each model, thereby yielding 4000 samples for each parameter tuple. Further details of all Bayesian models and their output can be found in the relevant sections of the respective scripts.

Besides the packages for Bayesian modelling, I made extensive use of the packages included in the *tidyverse* collection for performing data import, tidying, manipulation, visualisation, and programming in this book (Wickham et al. 2019).[1]

[1]The complete list of R packages used for analysis and visualisation is: *bayesplot* (Version 1.8.1; Gabry & Mahr 2022), *brms* (Version 2.15.0; Bürkner 2017), *cowplot* (Version 1.1.1; Wilke 2020), *effsize* (Version 0.8.1; Torchiano 2020), *ggridges* (Version 0.5.3; Wilke 2022), *tidybayes* (Version 3.0.0; Kay 2023), *tidyverse* (Version 1.3.1; Wickham et al. 2019), and *viridis* (Version 0.6.1; Garnier et al. 2023).

The original manuscript of this book was written within *RStudio* in RMarkdown format (Allaire et al. 2023) using the package *papaja* (Aust & Barth 2022). One of the key advantages of this approach is that all code and plain text is available within one single file for each chapter of the book and can easily be accessed and examined. All accompanying files, including raw data and RMarkdown files containing code and manuscripts, can be found in the *OSF* repository at https://osf.io/6vynj/ (and other repositories, as specified in the relevant chapters).

3 Intonation style

3.1 Introduction

In this part of the book, I focus on what I term intonation style, and on how it characterises the speech of autistic adults. The definition of intonation style is based on previous accounts of what the speech melody of certain speakers or groups of speakers "sounds like". If this sounds vague, it reflects the fact that there simply is no single unified account of how to define or quantify such global impressions of the prosodic characteristics of speech. Neither is there an established term that has consistently been used for the corresponding descriptions. I have chosen to refer to intonation styles, then, in an attempt to bring together insights from diverse accounts that share the aim of describing the prosodic features of speech mainly along the dimensions of liveliness and melodicity (a term used in related work by Hind 1999, 2002). I will pick up on the lack of consistent terminology again in discussing issues concerning the measurement and description of intonation styles in the following.

Intonation style has featured in research on autism starting with the very first descriptions in the 1940s. However, there is no clear consensus on what actually characterises the speech melody of autistic speakers. Also starting from the very first accounts, researchers have offered a vast range of mutually exclusive adjectives to account for what supposedly makes autistic intonation "atypical". These range from "robotic" or "monotonous" to "melodic" and "singsongy".

I will begin by reviewing the literature on the topic and in the process attempt to point out some reasons for this ambiguity. I suggest that, besides the underlying issue of the high degree of inter-individual variability in ASD, various factors are at play. These include the limited sample of the autistic population used in experimental studies (mostly English-speaking children), the methods used for eliciting speech (mostly unnatural) and the measures and analytical techniques employed (often vague or simplistic).

Following this, I present a novel method for capturing intonation styles and its application to the corpus of semi-spontaneous speech by 28 autistic and non-autistic German speakers investigated in this book. The results lend support to accounts describing a more melodic intonation style in ASD, but not to accounts describing a more monotonous intonation style.

I will conclude by summarising the results, putting them into a broader perspective and stating the limitations of the approach and the data at hand.

Parts of the background (§3.2) and an account of a prototype of the methodology described in the analysis (§3.3) have previously been published in Wehrle, Cangemi, et al. (2018), Wehrle et al. (2022). Key results presented in this chapter have been reported in Wehrle et al. (2020, 2022).

3.2 Background

At first glance, judging a speaker's intonation style seems to be a comparatively straightforward task. Listeners intuitively form impressions based on intonation, among other things, in many different contexts and without conscious effort. Putting such impressions into words with any degree of accuracy and confidence is a much more difficult task, however. This often results in the use of a very limited range of terms, with notions like robotic (i.e. flat or monotonous) or singsongy (i.e. lively or repeatedly spanning a large range) used as two endpoints of the same scale. An even greater challenge lies in the formation of scientifically testable operationalisations, which in itself presupposes the existence of measurements accurate enough to uncover the underlying features and parameters of intonation styles.

In §3.3, I present a novel method of measurement capable of reliably quantifying intonation styles. An application of this method to the speech data from the corpus of conversations between autistic and non-autistic speaker pairs analysed in this book is reported in §3.4.

In the following section, I will first give some background on the linguistic interest of intonation styles in general before examining the case of ASD in particular and pointing out methodological issues surrounding the description and measurement of intonation styles.

3.2.1 The linguistic interest of intonation styles

Intonation styles in general are of interest to linguists for a number of reasons. First, they are characteristic properties of individual speakers. Besides the character attributions formed in everyday spoken interaction, this facet of individual specificity is of interest from both a more practical and a more theoretical standpoint. Practical applications include forensic phonetics and emotion profiling (Ladd et al. 1985, Mohammadi et al. 2012). Regarding theory, the issue is pertinent both to the long-standing debate around the concept of idiolects (Paul 1880) and to the more recent, related debate about individual grammar networks (Cangemi et al. 2015).

Second, intonation styles are relevant for describing the behaviour of specific groups of individuals (within a language community). Intonation has featured particularly prominently in research on the speech of autistic persons (see Grice et al. 2023, McCann & Peppé 2003). Surveying previous work on the topic, there seems to be a broad consensus that many speakers with ASD produce "atypical" intonation. Quite what this means, however, and how it can be measured, is less clear. These issues will be discussed further in §3.2.2, dedicated to an in-depth discussion of intonation styles in ASD, and §3.2.3, focussing on methods and measurements that have been used to capture intonation style.

Third, intonation styles are also very relevant for the description of language varieties. There is abundant evidence for the influence of intonation styles on impressionistic judgements of different dialects. Data in Kuiper (1999: p. 258) show that Parisians consider the Provençal variety of French to be "singsongy", whereas they consider the Alsatian variety of French to be "jerky" (see also Nolan 2006). While it is always difficult to isolate such attributions from the wide range of cultural factors and stereotypes that may play a role, intonation styles in and of themselves are almost certain to be one crucial factor underlying such judgements. Intonation styles are in turn shaped by the phonological properties of the regional variety spoken. For instance, the varieties of French spoken in southern France are characterised by the production of clearly audible final schwas (mid central unstressed vowels) that would be much less prevalent in e.g. Parisian French (Durand 2010). This extends the segmental material available for the production of intonation contours and thereby provides an opportunity for more pitch movement (Grice et al. 2018, Torreira & Grice 2018). Although this phonological change does not necessarily lead to a more lively intonation style, it is likely to be one of the factors underlying the impression of singsonginess in this variety.

Fourth, intonation style is also related to the choice of register in speech. For instance, melodic intonation seems to be characteristic of infant-directed speech (IDS) (e.g. Holmes 2013). More melodic or even exaggerated intonation styles have been shown to correlate not only with better mother–infant bonding, but also with higher intelligibility and, as a consequence, with better language development in later life (Kuhl et al. 2008, Liu et al. 2003). Livelier pitch movement has furthermore been linked to speech by adults talking to (perceivedly) more attractive conversation partners (Leongómez et al. 2014). Why a more melodic intonation style might be used in such contexts is not entirely clear, but the choice of speech style in courtship is probably not orthogonal to experiences of, and positive associations with, IDS (as described above). More generally, lively intonation styles can be seen as indicative of evolutionarily desirable traits such as vitality and a lack of threat. Converging evidence can be found in studies reporting a *decreased* variability of fundamental frequency (f0) in conversational contexts marked by competition and high aggressiveness (Hodges-Simeon et al. 2010).

Finally, intonation styles are an important consideration in research on bilingual and second-language speech. It has been suggested that different languages can be described as, on the whole, having narrower or larger overall f0 ranges relative to one another. For instance, Dutch and Japanese have been shown to have an overall narrower f0 range than English while Swiss German and Norwegian have been shown to have an overall wider f0 range than English (Celce-Murcia et al. 1996, Graham 2014). Celce-Murcia et al. (1996) compare data describing the f0 range of English learners' various native languages (L1) with their productions of English as a second language (L2). Their results suggest that a speaker's f0 range in the respective L1 is transferred to the L2, with e.g. Dutch-accented English described as sounding "somehow flat" and Swiss-German-accented English said to have "a somewhat sing-songy quality" (Celce-Murcia et al. 1996: p. 193).

3.2.2 Intonation style in autism

As adumbrated above, the picture emerging from previous reports on intonation in ASD is far from conclusive. Quite remarkably, seemingly contradictory statements on intonation style in autistic speech even go back to the very first descriptions of autism. Sixteen pages into his landmark report, Kanner (1943) describes one of the 11 subjects portrayed, Herbert B. ("Case 7"), as uttering "sounds in a *monotonous singsong* manner" (Kanner 1943: p. 232; emphasis S. W.).

Similarly, Asperger (1944) in the original German refers four times to *Singsang* as characteristic of speech by the children he describes (pp. 87, 89, 93, 114), but equally notes that speech "proceeds...*monotonously*, without rising or falling" (p. 114; emphasis and translation S. W. – the standard English translation by Uta Frith does not capture this subtlety; cf. Asperger & Frith (1991) p. 70[1]).

While this descriptions might seem to be contradictory, it is important to remember that not only is the terminology used problematic (see below), but also that when describing more than one autistic individual, a high degree of variability should be all but expected. As we will see, apparent contradictions in

[1]Original: "[die Stimme] geht...monoton dahin, ohne Hebung und Senkung"

autism research often seem to be partly due to the related failures of 1) not adequately taking into account individual specificity and 2) not acknowledging the importance of the quintessential and intrinsic heterogeneity across the autism spectrum.

3.2.2.1 A note on terminology

The use of the terms monotonous and singsongy is problematic in itself, especially when these terms are used subjectively and without reference to any specific kind of measurement or rating scale. As the above quote from Kanner (1943) shows, the two terms might in fact be used to refer to one and the same intonation style.

The issue seems to lie mostly with the use of the term *monotonous*. This can be understood either as referring to a sameness of pitch, in the truly "robotic" sense, or as being simply unvarying, in a tedious manner (imagine the siren of a fire truck). This latter meaning is much more open to interpretation and is reminiscent of Kanner's description of a "monotonous singsong". Such an intonation style can then be imagined as being indeed singsongy, but in a stereotyped, repetitive manner, resolving the apparent contradiction. We also have to note that, quite problematically, the term singsongy can in fact be used with precisely and exclusively the above meaning, i.e. when it is taken to imply a repetitive melodic structure (often aided by rhythmic isochrony) that does not necessarily feature many changes in pitch. This stands in contrast to the usage in this chapter, where sinsonginess always implies a high degree of liveliness, melodicity and pitch dynamics. I will pick up on this terminological difficulty in Section 3.2.2.2.

Occasionally, the term *monotone* is used in place of monotonous. This usage seems to be more clearly with reference to a flat, robotic intonation style, but even here the dictionary definition is not unambiguous and allows for interpretations of sameness and tedium. In Section 3.2.3.2 I try to clarify the issue to some extent while introducing yet another closely related term, i.e. of a function being *monotonic* in the mathematical sense.

To add to the confusion (or possibly bearing a causal relation to it), all three terms – monotonous, monotone and monotonic – translate to the same word,*monoton*, in German. It is hence impossible to know precisely which nuance Asperger (1944) was aiming to convey in the excerpt cited above.

For the purposes of this book, I resign myself to using *monotonous* with the meaning of flat, unchanging pitch, in contrast to speech that is is *singsongy* in the sense of being melodic (or lively) and featuring many perceptible changes in pitch (occasionally substituting or adding the terms *robotic* or *monotonic* for reasons of style and clarity).

3.2.2.2 Evidence from previous research

In the following sections, I will take a closer look at some key studies describing intonation style in ASD. I will conclude by highlighting shared commonalities and contradictions in an attempt to identify possible causes for the lack of coherence and common conclusions. Please note that the vast majority of investigations into the communication of autistic individuals has been based on data from (English-speaking) children or adolescents, not (German-speaking) adults, as in the current work. Studies on intonation style are no exception. Accordingly, unless otherwise noted, the studies summarised in the following are based on data from (English-speaking) children or adolescents.

The following account is by no means intended to serve as an exhaustive review of prosody in ASD. For an in-depth and up-to-date overview,the interested reader is referred to Grice et al. (2023) and https://ifl.phil-fak.uni-koeln.de/phonetik/forschung/prosody-on-the-spectrum.

Evidence for melodic intonation styles in ASD

I will begin this survey with studies reporting more melodic intonation styles in autistic individuals. In total, such findings clearly outweigh those showing the opposite, i.e. a more monotonous intonation style in ASD. While claims to either effect have been made in the past, more recent research has quite clearly tipped the scales in favour of more melodic, not more monotonous, intonation styles as being characteristic of speech in ASD.

Simmons & Baltaxe (1975) found that speech in ASD is characterised by what could be described as more melodic intonation, or more specifically, speech with excessive pitch variation. They analysed the language of seven adolescents and young adults ranging in age from 14 to 21. There was no control group. The authors describe the speech elicitation process as "informal". The speech data elicited were clearly not spontaneous, however, as the autistic subjects, variously described as "isolated", "aggressive" or "naive" by the authors, were asked a set series of questions by (presumably) the experimenters, certainly by non-autistic adults unfamiliar to them. These questions ranged from the "informal", such as "Where do you live?", to the "abstract", such as "What do you think of the Vietnamese War?" (Simmons & Baltaxe 1975: p. 336–338).

Speech was analysed following the list of criteria used by Goldfarb et al. (1972), who investigated language in children with schizophrenia. The relevant criteria and the assessment are rather subjective (as acknowledged by Simmons & Baltaxe 1975) and wide-ranging. The most relevant criteria for our purposes are "excessive variation" of pitch level (see their Table II; p. 339) as well as "excessive pitch rise for stress", "excessive inflection" and "stereotyped (singsong)" intonation (see their Table III; p. 340). Simmons and Baltaxe ticked the boxes for all these criteria for the same four out of seven participants in their sample (probably reflecting the unclear distinction between some of these criteria in part). In sum, the study seems to show a trend for singsongy speech in ASD, but only for slightly more than half of all autistic participants – a pattern that, as we will see, mirrors the present findings in more ways than one.

In a more recent study, Nadig & Shaw (2012) report more melodic speech in the guise of expanded pitch range in a group of speakers diagnosed with ASD. They tested 15 autistic children aged 8 to 14, with 13 matched non-autistic children as a control group. Subjects were recorded in conversation with an unfamiliar adult research assistant in what is somewhat vaguely described as a "comfortable lab setting" (Nadig & Shaw 2012: p. 4).

The data used for acoustic analysis in the first part of the study is quite severely limited in both quantity and quality. The authors chose to analyse only "audio of the longest uninterrupted segment of each child's speech" (p. 5). Concretely, this means that for each individual only about 11 seconds of speech data was available. Additionally, this speech sample was by definition far from representative of participants' general speech style in being far longer than the average utterance. Nadig and Shaw do not provide information on average utterance duration in this part of the task, but in the later structured task that was part of the same study (see below), the average utterance duration was 2 seconds (comparable to the average IPU length of 1.4 seconds in the corpus analysed here).

The peculiar filtering of data performed by the authors is problematic not only as it entails excluding the vast majority of speech data recorded, but also because it is highly likely to have a direct bearing on the variable of interest (pitch range). Unusually long utterances can be expected to be produced with a more animated, lively speech style in general, and indeed a clear positive correlation between utterance length and melodicity was found in the corpus analysed in this book (see also De Moraes 1998, Cooper & Sorensen 1981). If we add to this the fact that sound was recorded through a single, ceiling-mounted microphone, leading to "sound quality [that] was not always ideal and sometimes contained environmental noise" (p. 5), it is not clear how valid any findings based on these data alone can be.

In any case, for this part of the experiment, Nadig & Shaw (2012) report a significantly higher pitch range for the ASD (median = 200 Hz) compared to the control group (median = 124 Hz). Mean values and standard deviations are not reported. Unfortunately, the data are also not available for inspection and independent corroboration. The authors report no difference between groups for mean pitch (mirroring the results reported here; see Section §3.4.3.2).

As a second part of the study, Nadig and Shaw ran subjective perceptual tests performed by non-autistic subjects listening to data from the first part of the study. Contrary to results from production, the perceptual ratings of both pitch range and mean pitch revealed no significant group differences. There was a significant difference only in ratings of "overall impression", which were given on a reduced, four-point Likert scale ranging from "normal" to "atypical".

Finally, the same autistic participants as in the first task were recorded performing a structured task. This task consisted of the children describing one out of four household objects. Compared to the first task, this yielded more and more varied data (8 to 15 utterances per child, with a mean duration of 2 seconds). However, ecological validity is a real concern in this particular setting, as the speech elicited was monologic and decidedly non-spontaneous. Similarly to the conversational data described above, results for this part of the task reveal a slightly higher mean pitch range for the autistic participants (156 Hz) compared to control participants (122 Hz), but no difference in mean pitch.

Despite the methodological shortcomings of parts of this work, the results in Nadig & Shaw (2012) reveal a clear tendency towards more melodic speech in ASD, and, crucially, do not give any indication whatsoever of the opposite, i.e. a robotic or monotonous intonation style.

Other studies providing evidence for an expanded pitch range in ASD include Fosnot & Jun (1999), Edelson et al. (2007), Hubbard & Trauner (2007), Diehl et al. (2009) on English as well as Sharda et al. (2010) on Hindi and Chan & To (2016) on Cantonese. I am not aware of any pertinent results on autistic speakers of German.

Evidence for monotonous intonation styles in ASD

Although some authors (including ourselves in previous work) have claimed that a monotonous speech style has in the past been generally assumed to be the typical intonation style for autistic speakers (Nadig & Shaw 2012, Wehrle, Cangemi, et al. 2018), closer investigation reveals that there is hardly any *unambiguous* evidence for this assertion. Take the pioneering work of Kanner (1943), which is often cited as an example for descriptions of monotonous speech in ASD. As pointed out above, the only direct reference to intonation here is the highly ambiguous description of utterances produced by an autistic child in a "monotonous singsong manner" (p. 232). What this use of "monotonous" here and in many other early studies (including Asperger 1944) seems to actually refer to is a general impression of repetitive or constrained behaviour (rather than a flat intonation style, specifically). Repetitiveness, however, can be just as much a part of a typically singsongy as of a typically monotonous speech style. In Kanner's concrete example, it probably refers to a speech style perceived as repetitive due to being particularly invariable or inflexible in nature.

I have indeed not been able to find any clear indications of a purely monotonous speech style in the literature, certainly not any based on pitch range or similar acoustic measures. However, there are some related findings that make claims to the same effect based on investigations of pitch accent choice and placement within the framework of autosegmental-metrical intonational phonology (Ladd 2008). Kaland et al. (2013) primarily investigated the intonational marking of contrastiveness by Dutch adults (not children as in all studies above) with and without a diagnosis of ASD, having elicited speech with a bingo-like game. The authors show that the productions of Dutch autistic adults are characterised by less variation in pitch accent types as well as a narrower pitch range, and that productions were judged by listeners to sound "less dynamic".

Despite some minor methodological issues, these results genuinely seem to reflect a more monotonous speech style in Dutch-speaking autistic adults. It is interesting to note that this study in particular stands out for not investigating the speech of either children or native English speakers. It is impossible to ascertain what role these factors might play without further work on adults and speakers of languages other than English. The results from the corpus investigated here, based on speech from adults speaking a closely related West Germanic language, however, do not support such an account of more monotonous speech in ASD in any way. Further, the work of Kaland et al. (2013) seems to stand alone in making such a claim, as all other studies that also find monotonous intonation in ASD simultaneously find evidence of singsongy intonation, as laid out below.

Evidence for both singsongy and monotonous intonation styles in ASD

In the following, I briefly summarise studies that show results consistent with *both* less melodic speech *and* more melodic speech in ASD within the same respective sample population.

Green & Tobin (2009) recorded 10 Hebrew-speaking children with and 10 Hebrew-speaking children without a diagnosis of ASD (see also Green 2009). The authors elicited both read and spontaneous speech. Results show that the ASD group as a whole had an extended pitch range compared to the control group.

However, typically for the inherent variability in ASD, the authors identified three distinct subgroups within the 10 ASD children: those with narrow, wide or, typical pitch range. This suggests that there were some individuals with more melodic speech and some with less melodic speech as compared to the control group.

Green and Tobin also carried out a categorical analysis in the tradition of autosegmental-metrical intonational phonology and ToBI annotation conventions (Beckman et al. 2006, Green & Tobin 2008). In this framework, the authors simultaneously found greater variation and a more repetitive use of pitch accent tones as well as a limited repertoire and more repetitive use of specific edge tones. This pattern is again consistent with both a more melodic and a more monotonous intonation style in ASD.

Thus, although results are not presented in exhaustive detail, it seems clear that both the acoustic and the phonological analysis in Green & Tobin (2009) suggest that ASD intonation style can be in line with control behaviour but also deviate towards either extreme, that is, towards a more melodic intonation style on the one hand and a more monotonous intonation style on the other. This is, again, indicative of the heterogeneity we can expect to find within any group of individuals diagnosed with ASD and also of the fact that we cannot expect communicative behaviour to reflect an idealised clear line of demarcation separating all participants with a diagnosis of ASD from all those without.

Other studies supporting the view that both more and less melodic speech can be found within a given sample of autistic speakers include Baltaxe (1984), Rapin (1991) and DePape et al. (2012).

Causes for conflicting results

There are at least three possible reasons for the uncertainty regarding the nature of intonation styles in ASD. First, the speech data used in previous studies were usually elicited through reading tasks, narrations, task-oriented conversation (as in this work) or structured interviews, none of which are guaranteed to yield examples of natural intonation (De Ruiter 2015, Grice et al. 1997, Spaniol et al. 2023, Kügler et al. 2015).

Second, as pointed out at various points above, speakers diagnosed with ASD constitute a very heterogeneous group, characterised by a high degree of individual variability. If speaker- and dyad-specific behaviour is not appropriately taken into account, as has all too often been the case in previous research in this and related fields, averaged values alone cannot be expected to paint a realistic picture of either the behaviour of the group as a whole or of any of the individuals within it (cf. Cangemi et al. 2016). A particularly important aspect of individual specificity in this particular case is that of age. The vast majority of previous studies only tested children or adolescents and/or featured very wide age ranges. This is not only problematic in itself, but also because, with age, many autistic individuals learn to employ compensation mechanisms in order to attenuate any behaviours that they have felt (or have been told) might make them appear unusual or conspicuously different from their non-autistic peers – but of course we neither can nor should assume that all autistic people indeed wish to camouflage such behaviours.

Third, where past research on intonation styles has gone beyond subjective impressions, it has often relied on vaguely defined and technically underspecified terms which do not stand up to rigorous empirical investigation. In the next section (§3.2.3), I aim to show that traditional measures are in principle not even capable of distinguishing stereotypical cases of robotic and singsongy speech.

To recap, despite the clear relevance of intonation styles to manifold aspects of language and to various levels of linguistic inquiry, the methods employed to measure, analyse and describe them have been far from uniform in past research. More importantly, it seems reasonable to question the adequacy of even the more common of such measures. To the best of my knowledge, there is nevertheless no (published) work dedicated specifically to tackling the issue of how to best quantify intonation styles. The current suggestions on how to ameliorate this situation were first described in Wehrle, Cangemi, et al. (2018), and I will summarise the approach in the following paragraphs.

3.2.3 Measuring intonation style: Past practice and new directions

While the characterisation of intonation styles has often been ill-defined and in the end achieved only through subjective listener judgements, there is a long tradition of studies investigating the closely related concept of pitch range (Ladd et al. 1985, Lehiste 1975). Together with the similarly widely used measure of mean f0 in the description of prosody, these measures form the core of a number of approaches that have aimed to capture the levels and fluctuations of a given speaker's minimum and maximum pitch values.

The most recent and widespread characterisation of pitch range can be found in the work of Mennen et al. (2012) and subsequent work by e.g. Urbani (2013) and Graham (2014). In this approach, pitch range is essentially described through a combination of linguistic and distributional parameters. This method will be critically analysed in the next section and followed by suggestions for how it may be complemented and refined, with the ultimate aim of better capturing and representing different kinds of intonation styles.

3.2.3.1 Linguistic measures

The idea of using so-called "linguistic measures" for determining pitch range originates with Ladd & Terken (1995) and is fleshed out in Patterson (2000). The key feature of this approach lies in the identification of "linguistically relevant landmarks" (Mennen et al. 2012) in the f0 contour. These landmarks are subsequently used in place of global, purely instrumentally determined minima or maxima for the calculation of a speaker's f0 range. In practice, this entails first reducing the f0 contour of a given utterance to a series of either high or low turning points. These points are then labelled as phonological tones, and averaged values are calculated within equivalent labels.

This approach has proven itself useful and yielded convincing results in the application to a number of different languages. Nevertheless, some aspects of the method suggest that there might be room for improvement in alternative approaches. For instance, the central operationalisation inherent in this method is rooted less in theoretical deliberations, but rather in purely pragmatic reasons, as pointed out by Mennen et al. (2012) themselves:

> Our decision to assume a direct relationship between turning points and phonological tones was driven by practical reasons so as to ensure consistency in our labelling. However, tones and turning points may not necessarily map in a one-to-one fashion, so that some tones may not be realized as turning points and some turning points may not constitute an underlying phonological tone (Mennen et al. 2012: footnote 3).

More importantly, the value and validity of intonational labels has come under increasing scrutiny and critical re-examination in recent years (see the contributions in D'Imperio et al. 2016). The method for measuring pitch range described above fundamentally relies on intonational labels, as they form the *starting point* for further analysis by providing a symbolic reduction of the continuous phonetic signal. This is consistent with a widespread approach in intonation research, used in studies from Hirst & Di Cristo (1998) to Hualde & Prieto (2016).

However, recent research strongly suggests that it might be more fruitful to take the opposite approach and use intonational labels only as the *outcome* of phonological analysis (Cangemi & Grice 2016, Frota 2016). In this approach, the use of phonological labels requires an evaluation of intonational meaning and of prosodic structure, rather than a discretisation of the phonetic signal. More recent developments go one step further by embracing this perspective while at the same time proposing a new method of analysis which promises to avoid many of the issues that are all but intrinsic to the practices of segmenting and labelling speech (Albert et al. 2018, Albert 2023, Cangemi et al. 2019).

3.2.3.2 Long-Term Distributional measures

The second pillar of the method employed by Mennen et al. (2012) (and others), besides turning points based on symbolic labels, takes the form of so-called "Long-Term Distributional" (LTD) measures. These measures are used to describe the range, mean, skewness and kurtosis of the distribution of f0 values. Using LTDs is an appropriate, even sophisticated way for describing pitch range, compared to earlier methods. LTDs are, however, still not ideal for exploring intonation styles, as illustrated in the following example.

Consider the f0 contour in Figure 3.1. This contour is stylised to the point that it would never be found in human speech data, but what it does give us is a useful idealisation of an f0 contour that would deserve the label *robotic*.

To show why LTDs are problematic for capturing intonation styles, compare the contour in Figure 3.1, which represents monotonous speech (and is monotonic in the mathematical sense, i.e. it never changes direction) with the one in Figure 3.2. This represents a stylised version of the other extreme: a thoroughly lively intonation style.

The crucial problem here is that these two very different contours yield exactly the same result in an analysis of LTD measures, as can be seen in Figure 3.3. An analysis relying on LTDs therefore obscures the polar nature of these two styles of intonation (at least in their hypothetical versions considered here).

3.2.4 Summary

I have shown that LTDs along with linguistic measures based on phonological labels cannot be considered satisfactory measurements for the characterisation of intonation styles. While a measure of pitch range should certainly be included, we need to also add a metric which truly captures the time-varying dynamics of pitch contours and is able to unambiguously distinguish (e.g.) the two very different speech styles exemplified in Figures 3.1 and 3.2. I will describe a two-dimensional analysis designed for this purpose, capturing both dynamics (*Wiggliness*) and pitch range (*Spaciousness*), in the following section.

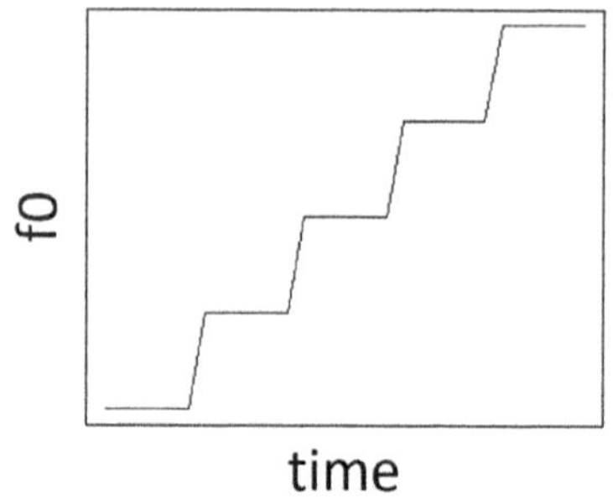

Figure 3.1: Hypothetical f0 contour of a monotonous (and monotonic) intonation style.

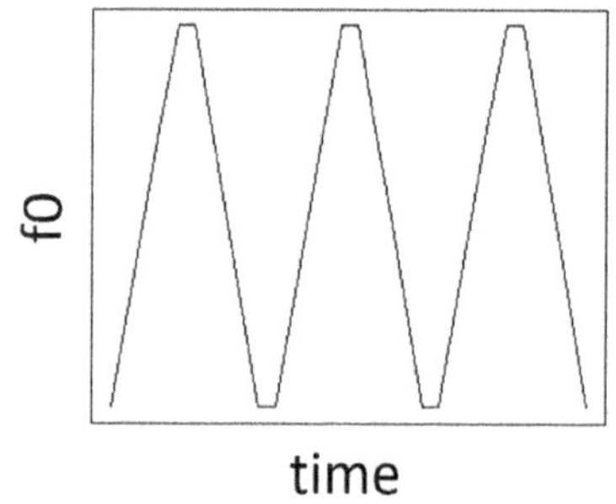

Figure 3.2: Hypothetical f0 contour of a lively intonation style.

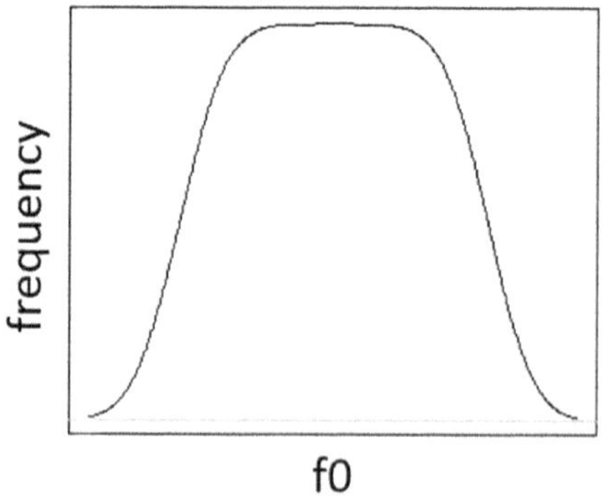

Figure 3.3: Frequency distribution (LTD) of both the monotonic f0 contour shown in Figure 3.1 and the lively f0 contour shown in Figure 3.2.

3.3 Analysis: Wiggliness and Spaciousness

The aim of the novel approach described here is to avoid the shortcomings inherent to approaches relying only on linguistic and Long-Term Distributional measures by concentrating on the time course and excursion of f0 trajectories. Two parameters are used to capture the melodicity of speech: Wiggliness and Spaciousness. The parameters are described in detail in the following. Since this approach was first described in Wehrle, Cangemi, et al. (2018), the method has seen 1) further improvement and automatisation; see the tutorial in Wehrle (2022), and 2) the successful application to an unrelated data set along with perceptual validation of the metrics used; see Wehrle & Sappok (2023).

3.3.1 Data

For the analysis of intonation style, all interpausal units (IPUs) with a duration of less than 1 second were excluded from further analysis, as such utterances cannot be guaranteed to contain enough speech material for a dynamic characterization of intonation styles. A large part of these short IPUs consisted of backchannels (listeners signals such as *mmhm* or *okay*) and filled pauses (hesitation signals such as *uhm*). The use of these specific discourse markers, including their prosodic realisation, is described separately in Chapter 5.

After the exclusion of very short IPUs, 4059 IPUs (with a mean duration of 2.67 seconds) remained for analysis. Any extreme values along all extracted parameters, as well as a number of randomly sampled IPUs, were hand-checked. After exclusion of any data points based on pitch tracking or processing errors, 4043 IPUs remained (> 99%).

An example IPU annotated with the relevant parameters is shown in Figure 3.4 and will be referred to throughout this chapter.

3.3.2 Processing

All pitch contours were extracted from individual IPUs (original extracted pitch contour represented as grey speckles in Figure 3.4), hand-corrected and smoothed (Cangemi 2015) (corrected and smoothed contour represented as a red line in Figure 3.4). The smoothed contours were then automatically stylised to a resolution of 2 semitones using the Manipulation function in *Praat* (Boersma & Weenink 2021) (stylised contour represented as a green line in Figure 3.4). By applying smoothing before stylisation, turning points are only located where an actual tonal movement is likely to be perceived.

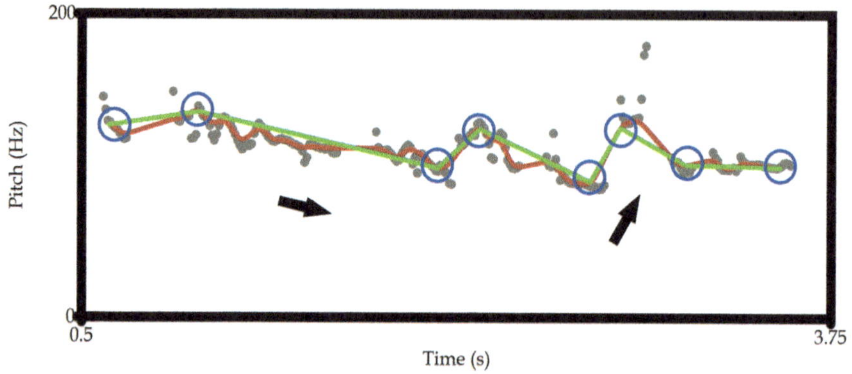

Figure 3.4: Representative example IPU with relevant parameters annotated. The grey speckles represent the original pitch track. The red line is the hand-corrected and smoothed pitch contour. The green line is the smoothed and corrected contour after stylisation to 2-semitone (ST) steps. The blue circles denote turning points in the stylised contour, used for calculating Wiggliness. The black arrows denote the two largest pitch excursions between turning points, used for calculating Spaciousness (see text for more details). This IPU has a Wiggliness value of 2.78 (8 turning points divided by a pitch duration of 2.88) and a Spaciousness value of 5.81 (average of the two largest excursions in ST), which is close to the respective mean values across groups.

Contours that have been smoothed and stylised at this resolution seem to be perceptually robust while also facilitating the further processing required to yield the final values of Wiggliness and Spaciousness. The threshold of 2 semitones for smoothing was chosen in Wehrle, Cangemi, et al. (2018) as an approximation for how intonation contours may be perceived auditorily. Careful experimentation has shown that the 2-semitone setting is a useful heuristic for capturing the essence of pitch contour dynamics. Moreover, the results reported in Wehrle & Sappok (2023) provide a first, highly promising perceptual validation for the chosen method. Comparison of a number of test utterances additionally revealed that *automatic* stylisation with a 2-semitone resolution, as performed here, leads to final contours that are very similar to the outcome of a *manual* procedure, as employed in e.g. Mennen et al. (2012), while being considerably more efficient. That being said, follow-up perception experiments are planned which may inform possible adjustments to the current method.

The additional steps necessary to yield the final characterisation of intonation styles along the two dimensions of Wiggliness and Spaciousness are laid out in the following sections.

3.3.3 Wiggliness

The term Wiggliness is borrowed from statistical analysis (see, for instance, Hall & Marron 1991). Wiggliness is operationalised as the amount of times an f0 contour changes direction in a given unit of speech (i.e. IPU) or, in other words, as slope changes per second. An automatic procedure was employed in *R* to compute the number of rises and falls within each stylised "Pitch object" in *Praat* (blue circles in Figure 3.4). This number was then divided by the total duration of the "Pitch object" to yield the final Wiggliness value. Wiggliness values ranged from 0.57 to 8.82 in the data set, with a mean value of 3.14 (SD = 1.07) across all IPUs.

3.3.4 Spaciousness

Spaciousness is operationalised as the extent of the slopes of individual f0 rises and falls within a given IPU, i.e. maximum f0 excursions. The final Spaciousness measure was automatically computed in *R* as the average between the absolute values of the two largest excursions (black arrows in Figure 3.4), calculated in semitones (ST). Spaciousness ranged from 0.01 ST to 15.63 ST in the data set, with a mean value of 6.03 ST (SD: 2.42) across all IPUs. Semitones (with a reference value of 1 Hz) were chosen for the calculation of Spaciousness rather than Hertz (originally used in Wehrle, Cangemi, et al. 2018) for being a unit of measurement that is much more closely linked to human auditory perception (Nolan 2003) and for additionally facilitating comparison between male and female speakers. A common reference level rather than one based on speaker means was chosen in order to obtain a more generalised and context-independent measure of melodicity.

3.3.5 Comparison with other measures

For comparison with measures used in previous studies, values of pitch range and mean f0 are also reported. Pitch range was calculated as the difference (in ST) between the maximum and minimum of (hand-corrected) f0 values in each IPU. The measure of ST was chosen over Hz here for the reasons laid out above regarding the measure of Spaciousness (i.e. perceptual validity and facilitated cross-gender comparison). This operationalisation of pitch range is in essence very similar to the Spaciousness measure introduced above, albeit less fine-grained. We can therefore expect results for pitch range and Spaciousness to be highly correlated.

Mean f0 was calculated as the average of all (checked and corrected) extracted f0 values from the speech of a given subject (total n = 658034) in Hertz (semitone measurements are not suitable for level measures; cf. Mennen et al. 2012).

The pilot results in Wehrle, Cangemi, et al. (2018) provide initial empirical evidence for the conceptual assumption that intonation styles described as more melodic are indeed accurately represented by *higher* values of both Wiggliness and Spaciousness and, conversely, that intonation styles described as more monotonous are accurately represented by *lower* values of both Wiggliness and Spaciousness. These assumptions are validated and strengthened by the analyses in Wehrle & Sappok (2023). It was further shown in Wehrle, Cangemi, et al. 2018 that the dimensions of Wiggliness and Spaciousness are highly correlated, but that each dimension contains some information that cannot be captured by the other. This observation, too, is firmly corroborated by the work reported in Wehrle & Sappok (2023). Wiggliness and Spaciousness can therefore be considered as complementary measures to a certain extent, and using them together rather than in isolation promises to yield a more accurate representation of intonation styles. Accordingly, the dimensions of Wiggliness and Spaciousness are considered, plotted and reported together, yielding a two-dimensional characterisation of intonation styles.

3.4 Results

I will first present overall results by group, then by speaker and finally with respect to speaker role, gender and dialogue stage.

3.4.1 Overall results by group

Figure 3.5 shows mean Wiggliness and Spaciousness values by group. See Table 3.1 for means and standard deviations (SD). The ASD group had higher Wiggliness and higher Spaciousness overall than the CTR group. The difference between groups is slightly greater for Wiggliness than for Spaciousness (as confirmed by Bayesian modelling, see below).

Bayesian analysis

Models for Wiggliness and Spaciousness were ran separately. Random intercepts for individual speakers were included in all models.

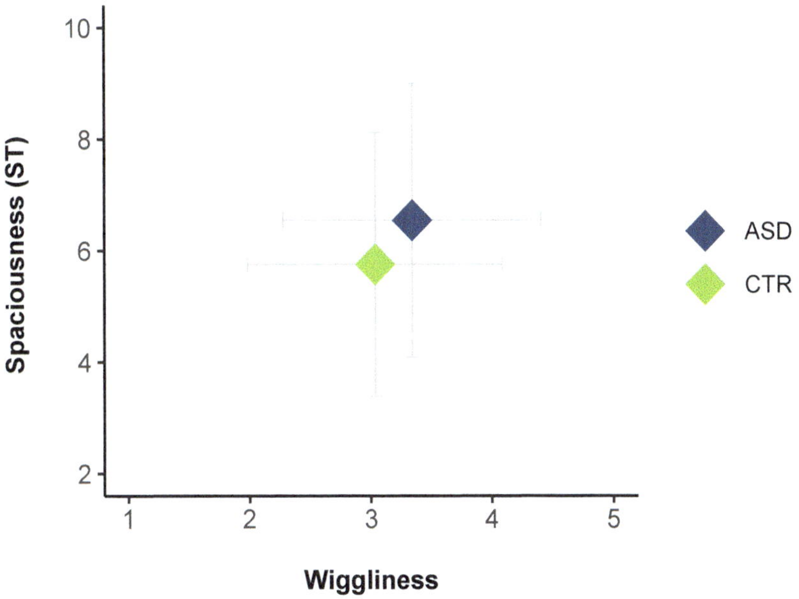

Figure 3.5: Mean Spaciousness (in ST, on the y-axis) and Wiggliness (on the x-axis) by group. ASD group in blue, CTR group in green. Error bars represent one standard deviation from the mean.

Table 3.1: Results by group (Spaciousness in ST).

	Wiggliness		Spaciousness	
	Mean	SD	Mean	SD
ASD	3.34	1.06	6.54	2.45
CTR	3.04	1.05	5.75	2.36

No effects of gender interacting with either Wiggliness or Spaciousness were found. Results will therefore be presented in models aggregating across male and female speakers (see the accompanying files and scripts for more detail).

Wiggliness

For the dimension of Wiggliness, the model output confirms that ASD speakers produced speech with higher Wiggliness ($\hat{\beta}$ = 3.45, CI = [3.25, 3.63]) than CTR speakers ($\hat{\beta}$ = 3.04, CI = [2.86, 3.22]).

Conversely, CTR speakers produced speech with lower Wiggliness – the group difference is presented from this latter perspective as the ASD group constitutes the reference level of the model by default. The estimated Wiggliness difference in the model is δ = -0.41, with a 95% CI of [-0.62, -0.19] and a posterior probability $P(\delta > 0) = 1$. This is evidence for a robust difference between groups.

The model used a skew normal distribution, as this provided a better fit to the data than a standard normal distribution. Regularising weakly informative priors with a normal distribution were specified for the Intercept ($\mu = 0, \delta = 6$) and for the regression coefficient ($\mu = 0, \delta = 2$). The default priors of the *brms* package were used for the shape parameter ($\alpha = 4$), the standard deviation of the likelihood function, Student's *t*-distribution ($\nu = 3, \mu = 0, \delta = 2.5$), and the standard deviations of random effects, Student's *t*-distribution ($\nu = 3, \mu = 0, \delta = 2.5$).

Spaciousness

For the dimension of Spaciousness, the model output confirms that ASD speakers produced speech with higher Spaciousness (measured in ST) ($\hat{\beta}$ = 6.79, CI = [6.25, 7.4]) than CTR speakers ($\hat{\beta}$ = 5.79, CI = [5.16, 6.34]).

Conversely, CTR speakers produced speech with lower Spaciousness – the group difference is presented from this latter perspective as the ASD group constitutes the reference level of the model by default. The estimated Spaciousness difference in the model was δ = -1.04, with a 95% CI of [-1.7, -0.38] and a posterior probability $P(\delta > 0) = 1$. This constitutes unambiguous evidence for a robust difference between groups.

The model used a skew normal distribution, as this provided a better fit to the data than a standard normal distribution. Weakly informative priors with a normal distribution were specified for the Intercept ($\mu = 0, \delta = 15$) and the regression coefficient ($\mu = 0, \delta = 4$). The default priors of the *brms* package were used for the shape parameter ($\alpha = 4$), the standard deviation of the likelihood function, Student's t-distribution ($\nu = 3$, $\mu = 0$, $\delta = 2.5$), and the standard deviations of random effects, Student's t-distribution ($\nu = 3$, $\mu = 0$, $\delta = 2.5$).

3.4.2 Overall results by speaker

Figure 3.6 presents results by speaker (and gender). This analysis reveals a considerable amount of individual-specific variation and a substantial degree of overlap underlying the between-group differences, although the overall tendency for higher Wiggliness and higher Spaciousness in the ASD group remains clear. The global impression of more singsongy speech in the ASD group is validated by the observation that both the five speakers with the highest mean Spaciousness values and the five speakers with the highest mean Wiggliness values were part of the ASD group. Conversely, the eight speakers with the lowest mean Spaciousness values and seven of the eight speakers with the lowest Wiggliness values were part of the CTR group (see Table A.1 in Appendix A for detailed results by speaker).

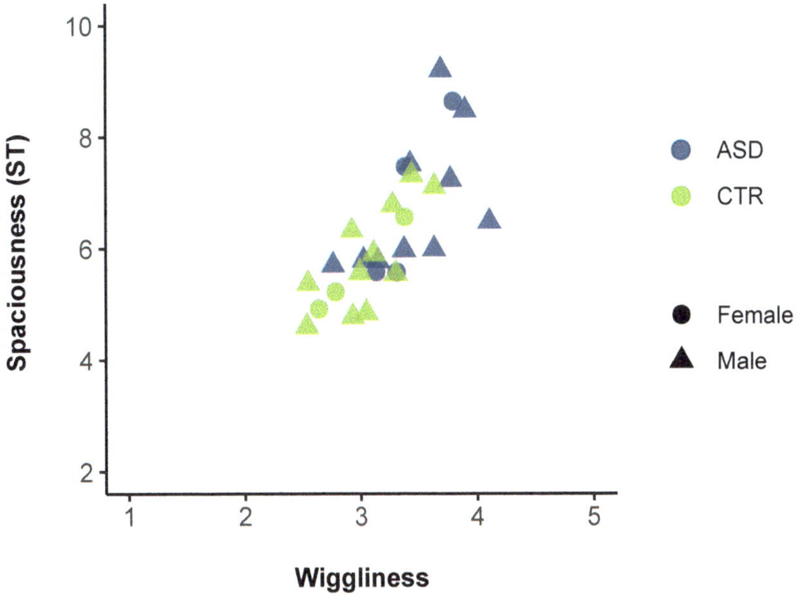

Figure 3.6: Mean Spaciousness (in ST, on the y-axis) and Wiggliness (on the x-axis) by speaker, group and gender. Circles represent females, triangles males. ASD group in blue, CTR group in green.

3.4.3 Comparison with pitch range and mean f0

For comparison with previous studies, the global measures of pitch range and mean f0 were calculated in addition to the novel measures described above.

3.4.3.1 Pitch range

Results for pitch range (in ST) are in line with the results for Wiggliness and Spaciousness by indicating a more melodic intonation style for ASD speakers, in the form of an extended pitch span (mean = 9.82 ST; SD = 4.09) as compared to CTR speakers (mean = 8.38 ST; SD = 3.78); see Figure 3.7.

Side-by-side comparison of Spaciousness and pitch range in semitones (as operationalised here) shows that, as expected, the two measures are very highly correlated (Pearson's $r = 0.99$).

A comparison of Spaciousness with pitch range measured in *Hertz* (rather than semitones) yielded a considerably lower correlation measure (Pearson's $r = 0.64$). More importantly, it was shown that an analysis based on the measure of pitch range in Hertz fails to clearly reveal the crucial between-group difference in intonation style, highlighting instead only the relatively obvious (and expected) separation of speakers by gender. This finding stands in contrast to results in Mennen et al. (2012), where only "marginally larger effect sizes for the span measures that were expressed on a ST (or ERB) scale compared to the corresponding Hz measures" are reported (for a data set of all-female speakers; p. 2256).

Figure 3.7 also serves to reiterate the crucial point that while there was a high degree of overlap between groups, about half of the speakers on the autism spectrum nevertheless clearly deviated from the intonation style of the CTR group (as can also be seen in Figure 3.6). These speakers produced higher values of pitch range and Spaciousness (as well as Wiggliness), indicating a more lively intonation style compared to control speakers.

The Bayesian analysis of pitch range confirms that ASD speakers produced speech with a wider pitch range ($\hat{\beta} = 10.32$, CI = [9.19, 11.34]) than CTR speakers ($\hat{\beta} = 8.45$, CI = [7.46, 9.43]) (measured in ST). Conversely, CTR speakers produced speech with a narrower pitch range – the group difference is presented from this latter perspective as the ASD group constitutes the reference level of the model by default. The estimated pitch range difference in the model was $\delta = -1.85$, with a 95% CI of [-2.98, -0.67] and a posterior probability of $P(\delta > 0) = 0.99$. This constitutes robust evidence for a group difference in pitch range. Further details on the Bayesian model can be found in the accompanying files and scripts (see https://osf.io/6vynj).

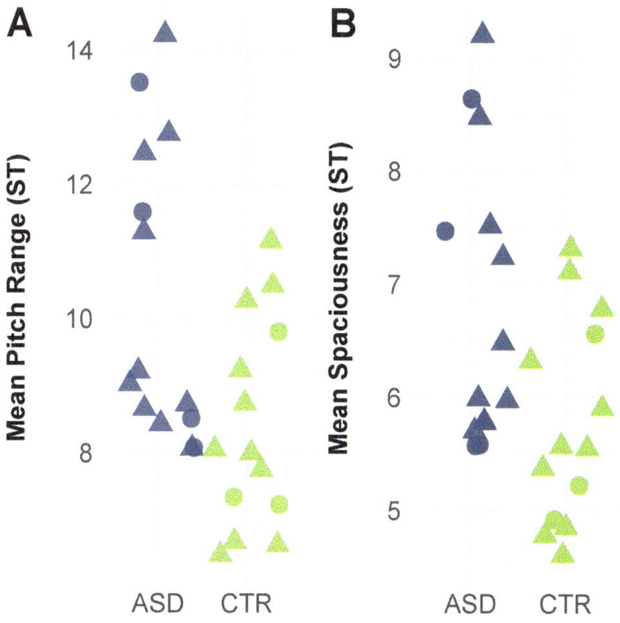

Figure 3.7: Mean pitch range (y-axis in Panel A) and Spaciousness (y-axis in Panel B) by speaker, group and gender. Circles represent females, triangles males. ASD group in blue, CTR group in green.

3.4.3.2 Mean f0

While both Spaciousness and pitch range, along with Wiggliness, have proven to be useful measures for analysing and displaying crucial features of intonation style, a comparison with mean f0 values reveals that this metric, although very commonly used in previous studies, is not sufficient to reveal the patterns described above. Mean f0 values are highly similar between groups, and a speaker-specific analysis does not reveal any meaningful underlying patterns; see Figure 3.8. See also Tables A.2 and A.3 in Appendix A for values by group, gender and speaker.

3.4.4 Effects of dialogue stage

Intonation styles were very stable across different parts of the dialogue (before, during and after discussion of the first Mismatch), with no clear differences whatsoever at the group level. A minority of speakers did show changes in Wiggliness

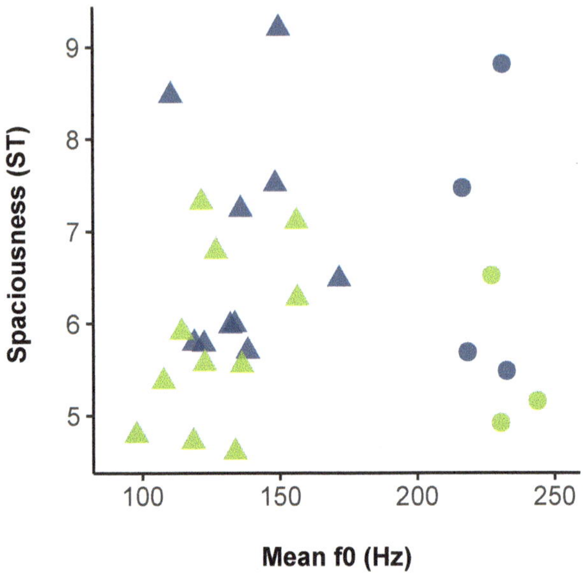

Figure 3.8: Mean Spaciousness (y-axis) and mean f0 (x-axis) values by speaker, group and gender. Circles represent females, triangles males. ASD group in blue, CTR group in green.

or Spaciousness values as the task progressed, but these changes were very subtle and not unidirectional. See Table 3.2 for values by group, and Table A.4 in Appendix A for values by speaker.

In the Bayesian analysis, models comparing early and remaining dialogue stages revealed estimates and 95% CIs around 0 and low posterior probabilities in the ASD group for both Wiggliness (δ = 0.03; 95% CI [-0.12, 0.19]; $P(\delta > 0)$ = 0.39) and Spaciousness (δ = -0.03; 95% CI [-0.37, 0.29]; $P(\delta > 0)$ = 0.55). The same is true for CTR speakers, with models for both Wiggliness (δ = 0.05; 95% CI [-0.19, 0.08]; $P(\delta > 0)$ = 0.75) and Spaciousness (δ = 0.04; 95% CI [-0.23, 0.33]; $P(\delta > 0)$ = 0.41) providing no evidence for a difference between dialogue stages. The models also clearly indicate no interaction between speaker group and stage of dialogue. Further details on Bayesian modelling can be found in the accompanying scripts and files.

These results strengthen the view that intonation styles can be considered as stable characteristics of speakers, differing considerably between individuals but proving robust across time and conversational context.

Table 3.2: Results by group and part of dialogue (before, during and after discussion of the first Mismatch). Spaciousness in ST.

		Wiggliness		Spaciousness	
	Mismatch 1	Mean	SD	Mean	SD
ASD	before	3.37	1.11	6.70	2.58
ASD	during	3.37	1.05	6.55	2.45
ASD	after	3.33	1.06	6.51	2.44
CTR	before	3.06	0.98	5.59	2.22
CTR	during	3.11	1.11	5.88	2.40
CTR	after	3.02	1.05	5.76	2.38

3.4.5 Effects of gender

Contrary to a speculative interpretation of the pilot data in Wehrle et al. (2020) suggesting that the difference between the ASD and the CTR group was less pronounced for female speakers, Bayesian modelling clearly shows that this was not the case. The data set was split by (self-reported) gender and differences for Wiggliness and Spaciousness were evaluated across groups (ASD/CTR) for each gender group. The resulting model estimates were nearly identical for the subsets for male and female speakers. For a complementary perspective, differences between male and female speakers were also analysed *within* groups. This confirmed that there was no gender difference in either the ASD or CTR group (e.g. the posterior probability in the ASD group was 0.43 for Wiggliness and 0.51 for Spaciousness; more details in the *OSF* repository at osf.io/gqe9n/).

3.4.6 Effects of speaker role

Comparing the roles of instruction giver and follower in the Map Task revealed a trend towards slightly more melodic speech by instruction givers across groups, as shown in Figure 3.9. However, the effect is clearer for the CTR compared to the ASD group. On average, ASD speakers produced higher Spaciousness in the role of instruction givers, but not higher Wiggliness; CTR speakers on the other hand on average produced both higher Spaciousness and higher Wiggliness as instruction givers.

In Bayesian terms, models comparing speaker roles for the ASD group clearly show that the speech of instruction givers was characterised by more Spacious-

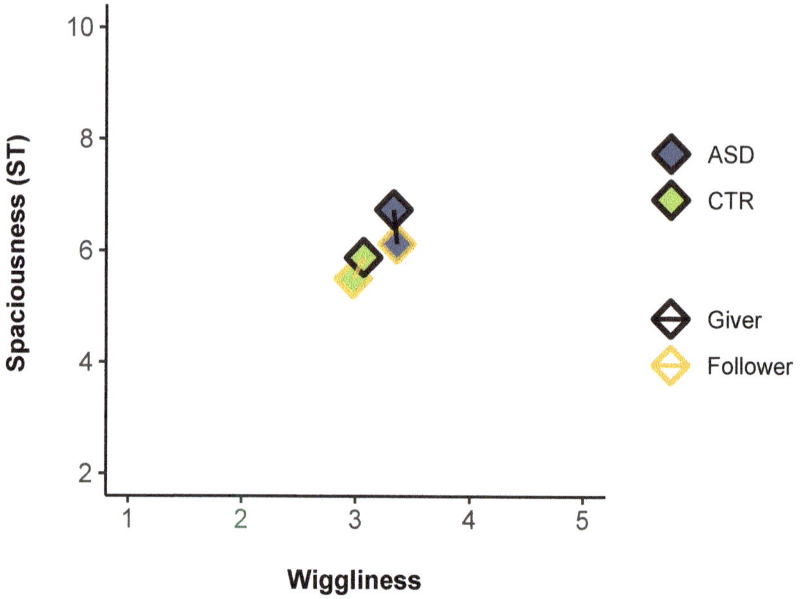

Figure 3.9: Intonation style by speaker role and group. Spaciousness (in ST) on the y-axis, Wiggliness on the x-axis. ASD group in blue, CTR group in green. Values for instruction givers are presented with a black outline, values for instruction followers with an orange outline.

ness (δ = 0.61; 95% CI [0.28, 0.95]; $P(\delta > 0) = 1$), but not by more Wiggliness (δ = -0.11; 95% CI [-0.3, 0.07]; $P(\delta > 0) = 0.16$).

For the CTR group, on the other hand, models comparing speaker roles confirm that there was both slightly more Wiggliness (δ = 0.18; 95% CI [0.01, 0.35]; $P(\delta > 0) = 0.96$) and more Spaciousness (δ = 0.64; 95% CI [0.35, 0.94]; $P(\delta > 0) = 1$) in the speech of instruction givers.

A speaker-specific analysis further reveals that the pattern of more melodic speech for instruction givers holds true for about half of the speakers within each group. In accordance with the group-level analysis, this pattern is, however, clearer for speakers in the CTR group (see Figure A.1 in Appendix A).

3.5 Discussion

The goal of this chapter was to appropriately measure, analyse and describe the intonation styles of autistic and non-autistic speakers. In order to achieve this, a novel method for capturing intonation styles using the two dimensions of Wiggliness (slope changes) and Spaciousness (pitch excursions) was outlined and then applied to a corpus of semi-structured dialogue.

3.5.1 Summary

Overall, a clear tendency for more melodic speech in the ASD compared to the CTR group was revealed. This tendency is evident for both parameters used, but the between-group difference is more pronounced for Wiggliness than for Spaciousness.

It is crucial, however, to expand on the simplifications inherent in any group-level analyses with a detailed investigation of speaker-specific behaviour, especially when working on data involving autistic persons. The speaker-specific analysis shows that group means accurately reflect the behaviour of speakers from both groups overall, but also highlights the fact that there is considerable overlap between speakers with and without a diagnosis of ASD. Half of the speakers from the ASD group (7 out of 14) produced a more melodic intonation style than any speaker from the control group, while the intonation style of the other 7 autistic speakers falls well within the range of values produced by non-autistic speakers.

It is important to note that where the behaviour of autistic speakers did differ from that of the CTR group, this happened only in the direction of more lively and melodic speech. It follows that the current study adds support to previous studies indicating a more melodic intonation style in ASD, but not to those describing monotonous or even robotic speech in ASD. Although findings on intonation style in ASD have been somewhat contradictory in the past, more recent studies have tended to find evidence only for more melodic speech (where differences were detected at all; see Section 3.2.2). This trend is corroborated by the results presented here.

One important caveat is that data from German-speaking adults were analysed. A comparison of the resulting findings is problematic in many ways, as results in the literature are overwhelmingly based on speech data from English-speaking participants, usually children. However, until we know more about the differences in behaviour of adults and children with ASD, or can make specific predictions about the interaction of autism with culture and language, this must remain a limitation which must be acknowledged but cannot be overcome. Overall, the fact that we now have converging experimental evidence from both children *and* adults, and from a range of different languages, strengthens the notion that there is a tendency towards more rather than less melodic speech in ASD.

3.5.2 Methodological aspects

A methodological comparison revealed that the patterns which were identified by using the dynamic characterisation of intonation styles along the two dimensions of Wiggliness and Spaciousness would not necessarily have been detected with the help of conventional linguistic and long-term distributional measures.

As pointed out above (§3.3), Wiggliness and Spaciousness are related measures. It is therefore not surprising that, in the current data set, speakers with relatively high (or low) values for Wiggliness usually also had relatively high (low) values for Spaciousness (and vice versa). This was not always the case, however. Speaker M08 (from the ASD group) has the highest mean Wiggliness value of all speakers, but a mean Spaciousness value that is very close to the group average. This underlines the importance of the *two-dimensional* approach to capturing intonation styles employed here (for further evidence supporting distinct functions and the partial independece of Wiggliness and Spaciousness, see Wehrle & Sappok 2023). Without reference to the novel measurement of Wiggliness, the intonation style of speaker M08 would have been falsely characterised as lying well within the range of intonation styles produced by control speakers and as being neither particularly monotonous nor melodic, when it in fact represents the *wiggliest* intonation style out of all 28 speakers.

Although the dimension of Wiggliness is conceptually related to what is known as macro-rhythm in prosodic typology (Jun 2012, 2014), its use as a metric and measurement is novel (but see also Kaland 2022, Prechtel 2023). Spaciousness, on the other hand, is essentially an analogue of pitch range, one of the most frequently used metrics in previous descriptions of intonation styles. I have shown that Spaciousness and pitch range values taken from the data set under study in this book are almost perfectly correlated. However, it is important to note that extensive correction and smoothing of *Praat*-extracted pitch tracks preceded any further analysis in this investigation. This level of rigour is not matched by all previous research in the field, particularly in cases where the authors' main expertise lay in fields other than acoustic phonetics (e.g. in the bulk of autism or second-language acquisition research). Therefore, pitch range as reported in previous studies is not necessarily a direct equivalent of pitch range as operationalised here. I am aiming to test, evaluate and adapt the measure of Spaciousness and to ultimately assess its usefulness beyond the established measure of pitch range in future work.

Potential adjustments notwithstanding, I have demonstrated the considerable methodological and conceptual proximity of pitch range and Spaciousness, and have have thereby shown that the proposed novel method of analysis is firmly anchored in more conventional, long-established research traditions and methodological approaches. This fundamentally strengthens the reliability and interpretability of the findings presented here and those of any future studies using the measurements of Wiggliness and Spaciousness.

In stark contrast, a comparison of Wiggliness and Spaciousness to mean f0, a measure very frequently used in previous research to characterise speakers or speaking styles, shows that an analysis relying solely on mean f0 would be unable to capture any of the patterns revealed using the measures described above. It follows that mean f0 is in fact not a suitable metric for capturing and characterising intonation styles, at least as defined here. Used in isolation, it seems to be too static and simplistic a metric to capture all of the complex, time-varying pitch dynamics that contribute to the perception of an intonation style as being more or less monotonous melodic. This fact does not, of course, invalidate any previous results relying on mean f0 for the description of intonation. It does strongly suggest, however, that more complex and comprehensive measures are needed to capture perceptual correlates of liveliness and melodicity.

3.5.3 Dialogue stage, gender, and speaker role

It was shown that intonation styles within speakers remain very stable across the duration of the recorded dialogue. This stands in contrast to findings from the same corpus showing that some other conversational behaviours, such as turn-timing and backchannelling, clearly differed between early and later stages of dialogue, particularly for the ASD group (see Chapter 4 and Chapter 5 for details). Intonation styles may therefore be considered as global, identifiable characteristics of a given speaker which are relatively independent of external factors such as interlocutor and conversational context. This invariance makes the identification of commonalities in intonation style across different individuals on the autism spectrum all the more relevant. Such common characteristics could ultimately serve as a kind of marker associated specifically with the language of at least some autistic speakers. Given the current results and those of recent research, a highly melodic intonation style seems to be a prime candidate for just such a pattern.

While no effect of gender was found, intonation style did seem to change subtly depending on speaker role. Speech tended to be more melodic for instruction givers overall, but this effect was more pronounced for speakers from the CTR group (who showed changes in both Wiggliness and Spaciousness, whereas speech in the ASD group did not change in Wiggliness). It might be speculated that CTR speakers were simply somewhat more flexible in adapting their conversational and intonational styles to their assigned roles than their autistic counterparts were. It is important to keep in mind, however, that the differences in intonation style according to speaker role were very small overall (for both groups). It is therefore not clear how robust or perceptually relevant these subtle changes might be in real-life interactions.

3.5.4 Limitations and implications

The data analysed and presented here strongly support the notion of a more melodic intonation style in (some) autistic speakers, while no support for the notion of robotic intonation in individuals with ASD was found. Any such claims will of course have to be tested in future studies on larger data sets of autistic and non-autistic speakers. Clearly, in a group of speakers as typically heterogeneous as that of individuals diagnosed with ASD, investigating 14 speakers will not be sufficient for drawing firm conclusions about the population as a whole.

Regarding methodological limitations, I acknowledge that although the comparison with conventional operationalisations of pitch range confirms the validity of the novel metrics used, the reliability (and potential advantages) of the two-dimensional Wiggliness/Spaciousness approach need to be critically tested and examined in future work. The main aim in such work will be to test how well Wiggliness and Spaciousness are aligned with listeners' subjective judgements of intonation styles. Some very reassuring first results from subsequent work can be found in Wehrle & Sappok (2023).

I will point out once more that previous studies on the same topic were performed almost exclusively using speech data from children and adolescents (or young adults). The results in this work provide a starting point for the characterisation of intonation styles in autistic adults, but it is important to keep in mind that results from children's speech will not necessarily be reflected in the speech of adults. In particular, it is likely that the relatively subtle group-differences shown here stem at least partly from the fact that many autistic speakers are able to adapt to the behaviours (including intonation style) of their non-autistic peers over time, if they so desire, in acts of social camouflaging (Hull et al. 2017, Lai et al. 2017).

This process may be aided by dedicated speech and language therapy, but such training is not a prerequisite for successful adaptation. With regard to the specific results and measurements presented here, it is entirely feasible that some autistic speakers in the sample may have been aware of having produced an unusually *monotonous* intonation style at some point in their lives and since learned to (over)compensate in producing a particularly *melodic* intonation style by the time of recording. Clearly, such speculations are not testable within the scope of the current data, but could be fruitfully considered as part of future longitudinal studies.

Furthermore, communication in the corpus under investigation was not fully natural or spontaneous. Task-oriented dialogue between autistic individuals (as in the Map Task paradigm) has to be considered as a major improvement on the read speech or formally constrained interactions between autistic speakers and non-autistic interlocutors that form the basis of most previous studies. However, there are also important limitations to the external validity of semi-structured dialogues as investigated in this book. Having to fulfil an unfamiliar task puts certain pressures and constraints on participants and the resulting linguistic output. This may have affected speakers in the ASD group differently than those in the CTR group. On the other hand, a restricted set of dialogue options and reduced chance of unexpected events should, if anything, suit the cognitive styles of autistic speakers more than fully free and spontaneous conversation. Combined with the fact that participants clearly formed part of the more socially motivated end of the autism spectrum, any differences between groups that were discovered in this study could be considered as all the more remarkable and meaningful.

4 Turn-taking

4.1 Introduction

In this chapter, we present experimental evidence on strategies of turn-taking in German adults with and without a diagnosis of autism spectrum disorder. Turn-taking is the most fundamental skill in spoken interaction and, although it is cognitively extremely demanding for interlocutors to exchange turns in quick succession, the timing of turn-taking has been shown to be remarkably fast in previous work (see references in §4.2.1 below). Rapid turn-timing has further been shown to be the preferred strategy by many different groups of speakers from varying linguistic and cultural backgrounds (e.g. Stivers et al. 2009). However, there is only scant empirical evidence on turn-taking in ASD and none whatsoever on turn-timing in conversations between autistic adults.

The results presented in this study constitute the first reliable quantitative evidence on the turn-taking and dialogue management strategies of individuals on the autism spectrum. Additionally, the findings on turn-taking in the CTR group constitute a major contribution to the thus-far relatively sparse empirical evidence on dialogue management in German in their own right. Data from Map Task dialogues performed by 28 speakers in disposition-matched dyads are presented. Turn-timing is investigated across the task as a whole as well as at different stages of dialogue, at both the group and the dyad level. Descriptive summary statistics, visualisation and Bayesian modelling were used to analyse results. Additionally, relative speaking times within dyads, prosodic aspects of turn-taking, and the effects of unexpectedness on turn-transitions are discussed.

For most aspects of dialogue management and when considering the dialogue as a whole, no differences between the ASD group and the CTR group were found. However, closer inspection reveals that 1) autistic dyads produced longer gaps between turns in the early stages of dialogue, 2) autistic dyads reacted differently to the introduction of matching and mismatching landmarks and 3) speaking times were less balanced within dyads for the ASD group. I will discuss the implications of these results, relate them to general theories of autism and to the notion of universal patterns of turn-timing in spoken dialogue, and furthermore compare the current findings with those from research on second-language speech.

The turn-timing analysis has been reported in Wehrle, Cangemi, et al. (2023), an earlier version of parts of the Match vs. Mismatch analysis in Janz (2019).

4.2 Background

Turn-taking is in essence a form of cooperative interaction. Humans engage in many temporally coordinated collaborative activities besides spoken interaction, such as manual labour, dancing or music-making (see e.g. Hawkins et al. 2013). Similarly, communicative turn-taking, in either the vocal or gestural modality, is not limited to humans. Many different species from different taxa perform tightly synchronised and regulated communicative interactions. Such behaviours are sometimes referred to with the term turn-taking in studies of animals, but behaviours described as *duetting* or *antiphonal calling/singing* can also be seen as equivalent to or even indistinguishable from what is often defined as turn-taking. For more details on the cross-species comparison, see Ravignani et al. (2019); for an overview, see Pika et al. (2018); and for detailed descriptions, see e.g. Takahashi et al. (2016) on marmosets and Fröhlich et al. (2016) on bonobos and chimpanzees.

Despite these cross-species similarities, human turn-taking in conversation seems to be a particularly remarkable phenomenon because 1) it is executed with split-second, even virtuoso precision and flexibility, 2) it involves the parallel prediction, planning and production of utterances which are improvised, yet rich with meaning, and 3) it is the key means through which human language, and to a considerable extent human culture, are learned and transmitted (cf. Schegloff 2020).

In the following section, I will first summarise the most relevant general research on turn-timing in human spoken interaction and then move to a critical discussion of previous research on turn-timing in ASD in particular.

4.2.1 General principles and patterns of turn-timing in spoken interaction

Turn-taking is the organisation of discourse into alternating units between speakers, with the aim of ensuring that generally no more or less than one participant speaks at any one time (Sacks et al. 1974). Most turns are short and most transitions between turns consist of very short gaps between speakers (Levinson 2016), which are preferred to other possible kinds of transition such as longer gaps or overlaps (two speakers talking at once).

A modal value of approximately 200 milliseconds of silence between speakers has been shown for a wide range of languages and speakers, with only slight language-specific variation (Heldner & Edlund 2010, Stivers et al. 2009, Weilhammer & Rabold 2003, Dingemanse & Liesenfeld 2022). This behaviour seems remarkably robust to individual, methodological and contextual variation – in contrast to many other aspects of language (Christiansen & Chater 2016, Evans & Levinson 2009, Schegloff 1989, Sterponi et al. 2015).

Effective turn-taking of precisely the kind described above is essential for the smooth flow of conversation, and human language is acquired, learned and practised almost entirely by means of these alternating exchanges of short bursts of speech. Gesture also plays an important role in the organisation of turn-taking, but as the methodology used to elicit speech for the corpus under study prevented participants from seeing each other, I will focus exclusively on spoken language in this account. For research on gesture and turn-taking in both signed and spoken languages, see e.g. McCleary & de Arantes Leite (2013), Holler et al. (2018), Zellers et al. (2016), Bohus & Horvitz (2010), De Marchena et al. (2019).

Although the smooth and rapid exchange of turns is so common in human interaction, starting with *proto-conversational* turn-taking in infancy (Gratier et al. 2015), it is cognitively extremely demanding. The fact that interlocutors consistently manage to avoid both long silent gaps and periods of overlap between speakers is quite remarkable given that the planning of even a very short utterance takes at the very least 500 ms and often considerably longer – 900 ms for utterances of more than two words, 1500 ms for simple sentences – far longer in any case than the well-attested typical short gap of around 200 ms (Gleitman et al. 2007, Griffin & Bock 2000, Schnur et al. 2006, Wesseling & van Son 2005).

It is therefore essential for interlocutors to *predict* the further content and the temporal endpoint of another speaker's turn, and to do so with a great degree of accuracy. This implies that interlocutors need to execute the cognitively highly challenging task of engaging in speech perception, planning and production in parallel. Although the interpretation of utterance-final prosodic cues is one important aspect of turn-taking, this in itself is not sufficient to enable the exchange of turns with sufficient speed and precision, as such cues appear far too late in the speech stream (Bögels & Torreira 2015, De Ruiter et al. 2006, Torreira & Bögels 2022). It seems most likely instead that a two-stage process takes place. In this account, interlocutors first plan and formulate (and update) their next utterance as early as possible in reaction to the message (predicted to be) conveyed by their conversational partner. This planned utterance is then stored in a kind of mental buffer until turn-final prosodic cues are detected in the speech stream of the interlocutor, at which point speech production is initiated (Barthel et al. 2017, 2016).

Prediction of a conversation partner's next utterance, at all levels of language, is therefore essential for achieving rapid turn-timing, and such predictions can only be made accurately if listeners are acutely aware of and attuned to the linguistic cues produced by their interlocutor.

4.2.2 Conversational turn-taking and autism

Differences in social interaction and communication are crucial criteria for diagnosing ASD. Among communicative skills, pragmatic aspects (e.g. inferring intentions and beliefs of a speaker) have conventionally been considered as particularly challenging for many autistic individuals, in contrast to more explicit aspects of language, such as syntax (Tager-Flusberg et al. 1990, 2005, Eigsti et al. 2007). A rapid exchange of turns requires certain skills which have been described in previous research to be "impaired" in ASD (Chasson & Jarosiewicz 2014). These skills include mutual perspective-taking and the ability to decode another person's emotional and linguistic signals.

Thus, it might seem plausible to assume resultant difficulties with turn-taking in the autistic population. However, the evidence is insufficient as only a small number of previous studies have investigated turn-timing in the context of ASD, and none have investigated conversations between autistic adults. Previous quantitative research on turn-timing in the context of ASD can be summarised most succinctly as reporting a tendency for more and longer silent gaps in conversations involving autistic individuals. The relevant studies are discussed in more detail in the following paragraphs.

In the first major empirical investigation into turn-taking in autism, Feldstein et al. (1982) report that 12 autistic adolescents and young adults (ages 14–20) produced longer pauses and shorter utterances (and therefore longer gaps) overall than controls, in line with previous, anecdotal observations reported in Fay & Schuler (1980). However, the generalisability of these results has to be questioned due to three key methodological issues: the age range and intellectual abilities of experimental subjects, the nature of the speech data under consideration, and the methods by which they were elicited (cf. Grice et al. 2023). The age range is such that at least some participants have to be assumed to be at different stages of language development, especially as this development tends to be delayed in ASD. Furthermore, no information is given on either general or verbal IQ. Finally, speech data consist of conversations between autistic subjects on the one side and either their parents or the experimenters themselves on the other side.

Therefore, by the admission of the authors themselves, "the interactions...were much more like interviews than unconstrained conversations" (Feldstein et al. 1982: p. 453).

More recently, Heeman et al. (2010) investigated 26 children diagnosed with ASD who were between 4 and 8 years old. All subjects were judged to be verbal and "high-functioning". Speech was recorded during administration of the Autism Diagnostic Observation schedule (ADOS, Lord et al. 2000), a standardised diagnostic test for ASD. The authors show that autistic children produced longer gaps than age-matched children without a diagnosis of ASD. However, the age (range) of participants and the method of elicitation alone are, each in their own right, reasons enough to preclude reliable conclusions on general strategies of turn-taking in ASD (for similar results on Korean see Choi & Lee 2013).

The authors of Warlaumont et al. (2010) investigated day-long naturalistic recordings between children and their parents and found longer silences before responses to questions in the ASD compared to a CTR group (see also Warlaumont et al. 2014).

The most recent published work of relevance (Ochi et al. 2019) is notable for featuring adult autistic participants, although they were considerably younger on average than in the sample under investigation in this book. Speech data were limited to recordings of the ADOS schedule. Similarly to all the above studies, Ochi et al. (2019) found a clear tendency for longer silent gaps in the ASD compared to a control group.

Finally, in a meta-analysis of the literature on adult–infant turn-taking, Nguyen et al. (2022) confirm the overall trend for more and longer between-turn silences in conversations involving individuals on the autism spectrum.

One notable departure from this consensus can be found in the wide-ranging and influential "anthropological perspective" put forward in Ochs et al. (2004). The authors set out to understand autistic persons not as isolated individuals but rather as social actors with a diverse range of strengths and difficulties in relation to socio-cultural factors and expectations. Crucially, in describing a "cline of competence" across different social domains, Ochs et al. (2004) report that in the domain of conversational turn-taking, autistic children show few difficulties and "seem to behave qualitatively like many of the unaffected [sic] peers in their families and communities" (p. 162). They speculate that the "local orderliness of sequences" might suit the cognitive style typical for persons on the autism spectrum. The quantitative findings on autistic adults from this work, revealing no clear overall differences in turn-timing between the ASD and the CTR group, add some support to this earlier qualitative account.

4.3 Data and analysis

Speech data from 28 German-speaking adults, 14 with and 14 without a diagnosis of ASD, were analysed. Speakers were recorded in disposition-matched dyads (ASD–ASD; CTR–CTR). For further details on subjects and materials, see Chapter 2.

The data set under study contains 18332 IPUs in total (inter-pausal units; here defined as speech separated by at least 200 milliseconds of silence). For an analysis of turn-taking, not these units of speech in themselves are of primary interest, but rather the points of transition between them. The data set contains 5668 such transitions overall. There are fewer turn transitions than IPUs because most of the latter were followed by another IPU from the same speaker; i.e. separated by within-speaker pauses (see §5.5) rather than between-speaker gaps.

The start and end points of all transitions were precisely labelled by hand following an automatic first-pass segmentation of recordings into silent and non-silent intervals using *Praat* (version 6.1.09) (Boersma & Weenink 2021). I broadly follow the methodology of Levinson & Torreira (2015) – which in turn builds on Heldner & Edlund (2010) – for the continuous analysis of turn-timing, in order to facilitate comparison of the current results to previous work. Accordingly, audible in-breaths, clicks and similar noises were counted as part of *silent* intervals, rather than speech. Filled pauses such as *uhm*, on the other hand, were annotated as being part of non-silent utterances. Thus, I followed the approach of essentially analysing turn-timing from a linguistic, rather than a purely acoustic perspective (which would incidentally not solve the problem of experimenters having to subjectively determine thresholds for what is considered silence).

Following Levinson & Torreira (2015), all turn transitions were categorised as being either *gaps*, *between-overlaps* or *within-overlaps*; see definitions in Figure 4.1. Within-overlaps do *not* in fact entail a floor transfer from one speaker to another, and did therefore not enter into the analysis of turn-timing. Distribution and characteristics of within-overlaps are instead discussed separately in §4.4.4.1.

Of the 5668 transitions in the data set, 3418 were silent gaps (60.3%), 1326 were between-overlaps (23.3%) and 924 were within-overlaps (16.3%). After the exclusion of within-overlaps, 4744 transitions remained for the analysis of turn-timing. Of these, 72% were gaps, and 28% were (between-)overlaps.

I follow previous studies on turn-timing in analysing turn transitions using the measure of Floor Transfer Offset (FTO), in which positive values represent gaps and negative values represent overlaps between speakers. Figure 4.2 gives a schematic representation.

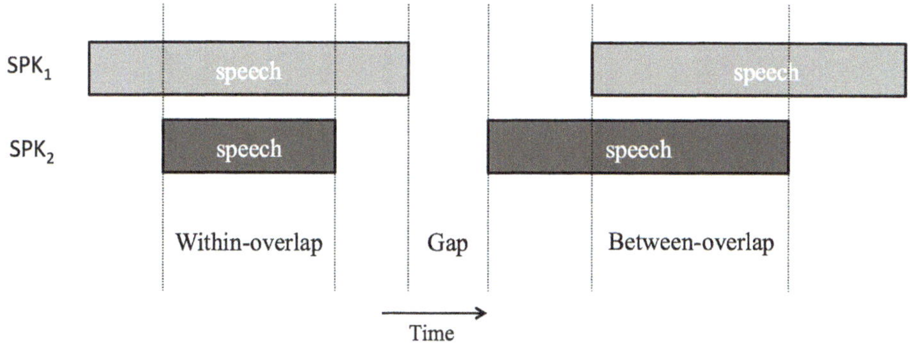

Figure 4.1: Categories of turn transition (adapted from Levinson & Torreira 2015). *Gaps* are silent intervals between turn transitions; *between-overlaps* are turn transitions composed of overlapping speech from both interlocutors. *Within-overlaps* are not true floor transfer transitions, but rather represent passages of overlapping speech which are *not* followed by a change of speaker (and therefore did not enter into turn-timing analyses). SPK = Speaker.

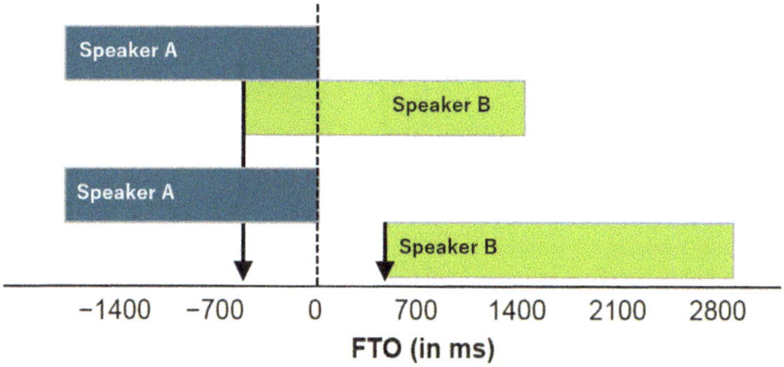

Figure 4.2: Floor Transfer Offset (FTO) measurements: Overlaps are represented with negative FTO values (see left arrow for an FTO value of about -600 ms); gaps are represented with positive FTO values (see right arrow for an FTO value of about +600 ms).

Bayesian linear modelling was used to test for group differences in FTO values (with DYAD as a random factor). Further, the interaction of FTO values with part of dialogue (see §4.4.1.3 for details) was tested in order to examine whether temporal dynamics might reveal any ASD-specific patterns.

Bayesian modelling confirmed that, across groups, there was no difference in FTO between all-male, all-female and mixed dyads. Gender as a factor was therefore disregarded in the following analyses.[1]

4.4 Results

I will first present the overall results on turn-timing in a continuous analysis. Results are presented at the level of groups as well as dyads and include an analysis taking into account different dialogue stages. The continuous analysis is complemented by a categorical analysis of different transition types.

This is followed by an in-depth analysis examining the role of unexpectedness in turn-timing. All transitions directly following the introduction of new landmarks were compared, contrasting Matches and Mismatches.

Finally, dialogue patterns beyond turn transitions are considered with an investigation of the overall distribution of silence, single-speaker speech and overlapping speech. Further, speaking times within dyads are compared, an overview visualisation of all turns for all dyads is presented, and an exploratory analysis of the prosodic constructions used to mark turn-ends and turn-beginnings is outlined.

4.4.1 Continuous analysis of turn transitions

The following results are presented using the measure of Floor Transfer Offset (FTO), which allows for a continuous representation of both gaps and overlaps along the same dimension by representing gaps between speakers as positive values and overlaps as negative values.

4.4.1.1 Overall results by group

Figure 4.3 shows turn-timing values by group. Visual inspection alone makes it clear that values are very similar across groups. Overall, the ASD group has

[1] A Gaussian model with FLOOR TRANSFER OFFSET as the dependent variable, GENDER COMBINATION (all-female/all-male/mixed) as a fixed factor and DYAD as a random factor was used, and no robust differences between any of the groups was found – more details in the accompanying *OSF* repository at https://osf.io/v5pn4/.

slightly higher FTO values, with a mean of 317 ms (SD: 599) and a median of 205 ms, compared to the CTR group with a mean of 238 ms (SD: 555) and a median of 175 ms.

Assuming 100-millisecond bins, both the ASD and the CTR group have a modal FTO value of 200 ms. In this regard, the current study directly replicates a number of previous findings on turn-timing from Stivers et al. (2009) onwards. Figure B.1 in Appendix B presents histograms using 100-millisecond bins and is directly modelled after the histograms presented in Levinson & Torreira (2015).

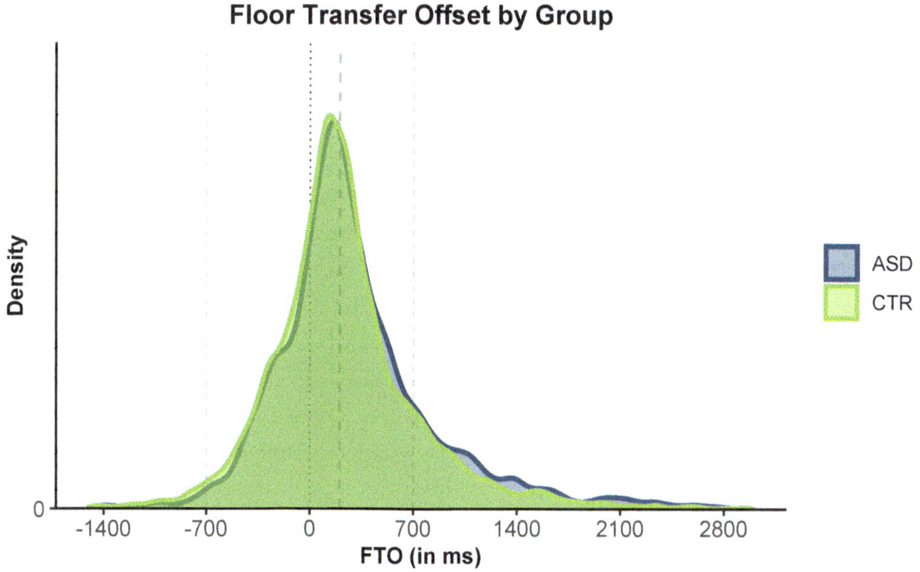

Figure 4.3: Floor Transfer Offset (FTO) values by group. Positive values represent gaps; negative values represent overlaps. ASD group in blue, CTR group in green. The dotted line indicates the value of 0 ms FTO, representing no-gap-no-overlap transitions. Dashed lines indicate the values of +200 ms (expected for typical transitions) and +/-700 ms FTO (unusually long transitions).

Bayesian analysis

A Gaussian model with FTO as the dependent variable, GROUP (ASD/CTR) as a fixed factor and DYAD as a random factor was used for Bayesian analysis (more details below and in the accompanying files).

Model output confirms that ASD dyads produced somewhat higher FTO values (in ms) ($\hat{\beta}$ = 326, 95% CI = [237, 414]) than CTR speakers ($\hat{\beta}$ = 250, 95% CI = [174, 337]). The group difference in the model is reported with the ASD group as the reference level. Mean δ = -74, indicating a trend towards lower FTO values in the CTR group. However, the 95% CI [-173, 25] includes zero by some margin and the posterior probability $P(\delta > 0) = 0.9$ is below the heuristic threshold of 0.95. The model therefore does not suggest a reliable difference between groups, only a trend towards higher FTO values (i.e. longer gaps) in autistic dyads.

A model with a normal distribution was used, and weakly informative priors with a normal distribution were specified for the intercept (μ = 0, δ = 6000) and for the regression coefficient (μ = 0, δ = 1000). The default priors of the *brms* package were used for the standard deviation of the likelihood function, namely a Student's *t*-distribution (ν = 3, μ = 0, δ = 363.2), and for the standard deviations of random effects, Student's *t*-distribution (ν = 3, μ = 0, δ = 363.2).

4.4.1.2 Overall results by dyad

Figure 4.4 presents FTO values by dyad. The plot clearly shows that distributions are extremely similar across dyads. Note, for instance, that the dashed line at the 200 ms mark (indicating very short gaps) runs close to the distributional peak of all dyads from both groups. Assuming a bin width of 100 milliseconds, 11 out of all 14 dyads produced a modal value of 200 ms (with the modes of the remaining dyads not deviating by more than 100 ms). Mean FTO values ranged from 137 ms to 503 ms across dyads. The group-level tendency towards slightly higher FTO values in the ASD group is reflected in the fact that four out of the five highest mean FTO values were produced by ASD dyads and four out of the five lowest mean values were produced by CTR dyads.

In order to corroborate the representativeness of group-level results, it was tested whether any single dyad had a decisive influence on the group level patterns by successively omitting individual dyads and rerunning the group-level analysis, and this was found not to be the case.

4.4.1.3 Results by dialogue stage

Although the turn-timing behaviours of the ASD and the CTR group were quite similar overall, some clear differences between groups are revealed when we do not only consider FTO results across the dialogue as a whole, but also compare early with later dialogue stages. Detection of the first Mismatch in the first Map Task is used as a cut-off point: all dialogue preceding detection is counted as being part of the beginning of the conversation, all dialogue following detection as the remainder of the conversation (more details in §2.2, §4.4.1.4 and §4.4.4.4).

Figure 4.5 shows FTO values by group and dialogue stage. While autistic dyads performed turn-timing essentially equivalent to that of non-autistic dyads for

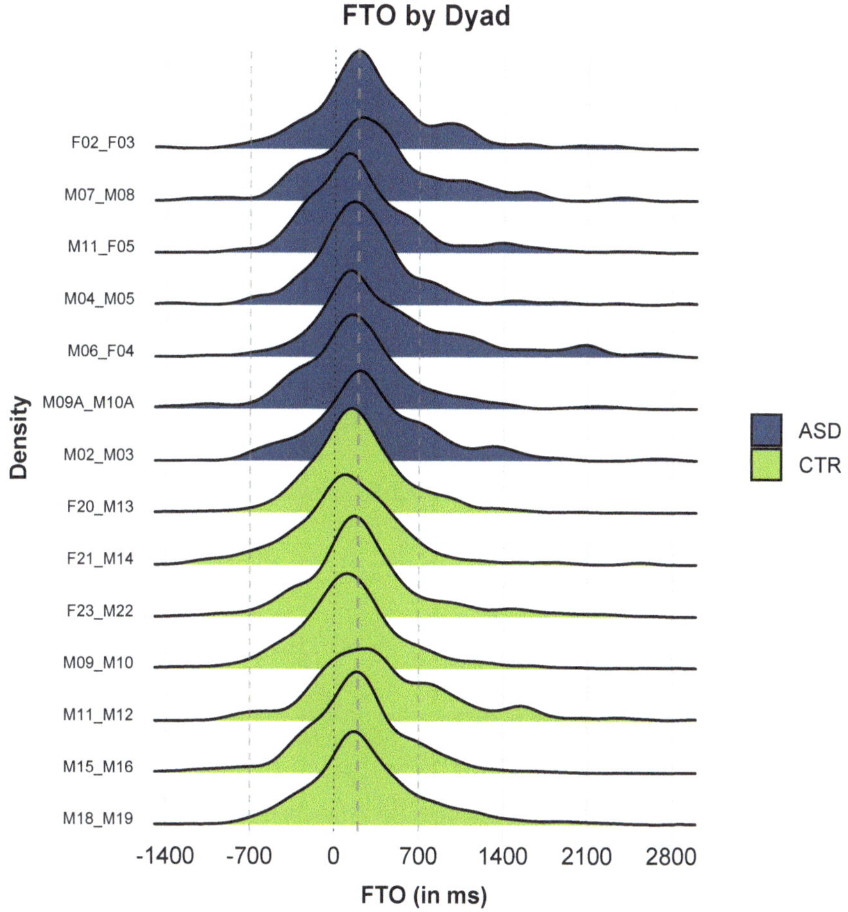

Figure 4.4: Floor Transfer Offset (FTO) values by dyad. Positive values represent gaps; negative values represent overlaps. ASD group in blue, CTR group in green.

most of the dialogue, they did not arrive at this timing instantly. In fact, during the first few minutes of dialogue, before the first Mismatch in the Map Task was detected (2 minutes or 10% of overall duration into the task on average), FTO values for the ASD group were far higher (mean = 511 ms; SD = 799) than in the remainder of the dialogue (mean = 299 ms; SD = 576). These values indicate considerably longer silent gaps between ASD dyads early in the task. Dyads in the CTR group show only a slight change, and in the opposite direction, with shorter gaps (and slightly more overlaps) in the beginning of the dialogue (mean = 191 ms; SD = 540) compared to the remainder (mean = 243 ms; SD = 558). This interaction signifies that the turn-timing behaviour of the CTR and the ASD group differed considerably in the beginning of conversations (δ = 320 ms), but not at later stages (δ = 56 ms).

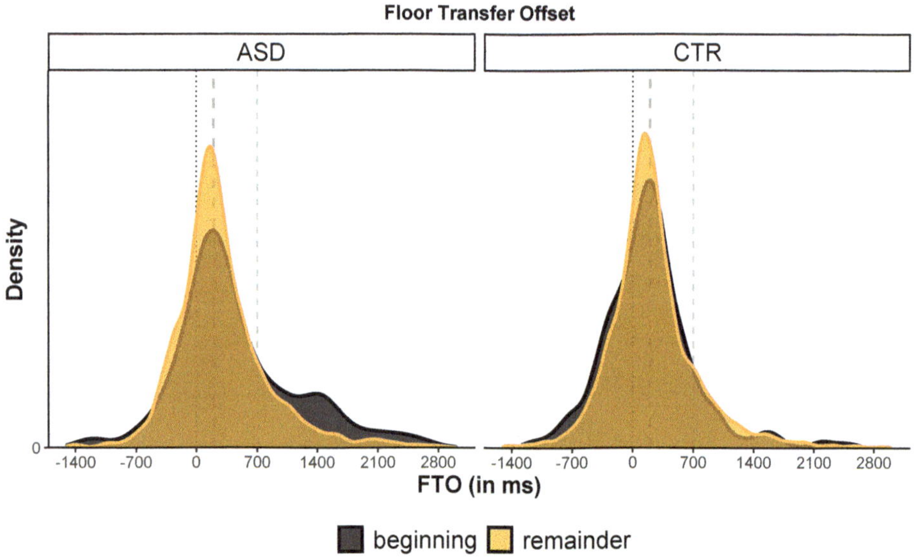

Figure 4.5: FTO values by group and dialogue stage. The black curve represents the beginning of the dialogue (until detection of the first Mismatch); the orange curve represents the remainder of the dialogue (after detection of the first Mismatch). Positive values represent gaps; negative values represent overlaps. ASD group on the left, CTR group on the right.

Figure 4.6 presents FTO values by dialogue stage and dyad, with CTR dyads in the top half of the plot and ASD dyads in the bottom half. We can see that for most (but not all) CTR dyads, FTO values were essentially the same for early and later stages of dialogue. For most (but not all) ASD dyads, on the other hand, there was a lot of variability in the early stages of dialogue, mostly (but not only) in the direction of longer gaps. This variability disappeared after the initial stages, as the dyads seemed to settle into a temporally stable turn-taking style that is virtually indistinguishable from that of CTR dyads.

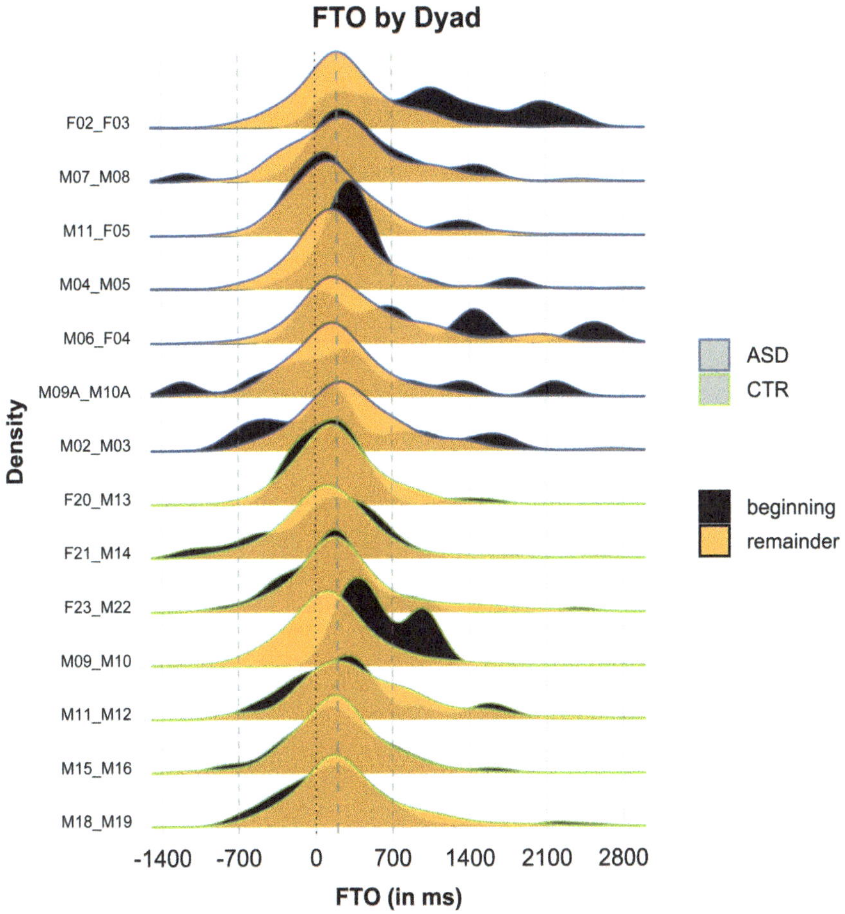

Figure 4.6: Floor Transfer Offset (FTO) values by dialogue stage and dyad. Positive values represent gaps; negative values represent overlaps. ASD dyads in the top half and outlined in blue, CTR dyads in the bottom half and outlined in green. Black curves represent the beginning of dialogue (before detection of the first Mismatch); orange curves represent the remaining dialogue (after detection of the first Mismatch).

4.4.1.4 Corroboration of dialogue stage effect

For the analyses reported directly above, detection (i.e. first mention) rather than resolution of the first Mismatch (i.e. the time when interlocutors finished discussing the first Mismatch and moved on to the remainder of the task) was used as a cut-off point for the early stages of dialogue. There are two main reasons for this choice. First, a detailed analysis of all turn transitions directly following the introduction of matching vs. mismatching landmarks reveals that there was a consistent and distinct reaction to the detection of the first Mismatch in both groups (in the form of longer gaps). For details see §4.4.3; see also Janz (2019). Essentially, the first Mismatch can thus be seen as a turning point in the interaction. Before detection of the first Mismatch, participants might feel that they are expected to give their individual contribution to the solution of a known problem (i.e. draw a path on an otherwise identical map). After the first Mismatch is detected, participants might feel that they need to give a joint contribution to navigate an unknown problem (knowing that the two maps are not identical), and this difference in the conversational goal can be expected to generate a difference in the interaction.

The second reason for using detection rather than resolution is that the former is less problematic as a timestamp from a practical perspective. The time it took to resolve the first Mismatch varied widely across dyads, ranging in duration from under 10 seconds to over 5 minutes. Moreover, even determining when a Mismatch was in fact resolved can be difficult and involves a degree of subjective judgement. In contrast, the detection of the first Mismatch was in almost all cases unambiguously expressed directly in the speech of both interlocutors.

To conclusively examine the appropriateness of using detection of the first Mismatch as the cut-off point, two further analyses were performed: 1) a further analysis taking into account the three-way distinction of a) dialogue from the start of the task to the detection of the first Mismatch, b) dialogue during the discussion and up to the resolution of the first Mismatch and c) all remaining (following) dialogue, and 2) a continuous analysis of FTO values in the first 100 turn transitions.

Briefly, the analysis with a three-way distinction of dialogue stages confirms that there was a robust between-group difference only before detection, not during and after the discussion of the first Mismatch (details of statistical modelling are reported in the following section).

Finally, Figure 4.7 shows that average FTO values in the ASD group tended to continuously decrease from the start of conversations until the point when the first Mismatch was detected, strengthening the validity of using mismatch detection as a cut-off point. Note that Figure 4.7 shows only the first 100 turn transitions; dialogues contained a total of 400 transitions on average.

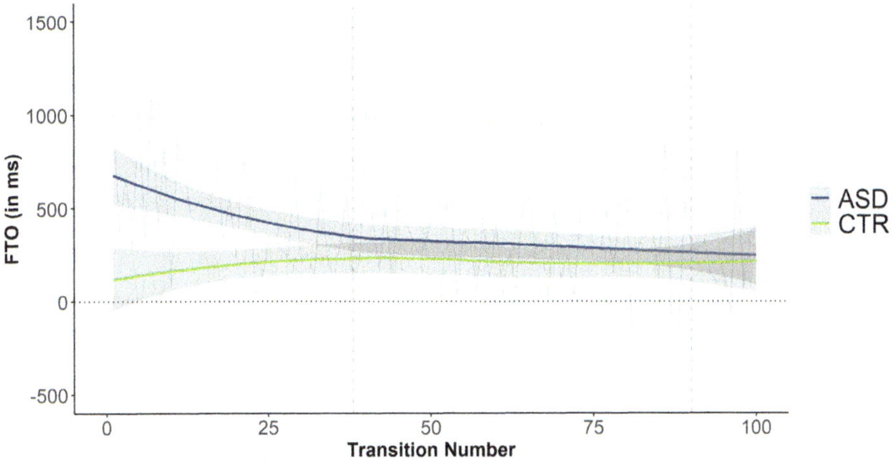

Figure 4.7: FTO values by turn transition and group. Positive values represent gaps; negative values represent overlaps. ASD group in blue, CTR group in green. Thin blue/green lines represent averaged FTO values by transition and group; thick lines represent fitted LOESS-smoothed curves by group, the surrounding grey shaded areas the respective standard error. The dashed vertical lines show 1) transition no. 38 (average time point for detection of first Mismatch) and 2) transition no. 90 (average time point for resolution of first Mismatch).

We can conclude that differences in turn-timing were indeed greater between groups in the early stages of dialogue compared to the remainder, independent of the specific cut-off point.

Bayesian analysis

Bayesian modelling confirms the above description in showing that there was a clear difference in FTO between groups early on in the dialogue, but not at later stages. More details on the interaction between group (CTR vs. ASD) and dialogue stage are given below.

Group differences are reported with the ASD group as the reference level and differences between dialogue stages are reported with the beginning of the dialogue as the reference level. First, a Gaussian model with FTO as the dependent variable, the interaction GROUP (ASD/CTR)*DIALOGUE STAGE (before/after detection of the first Mismatch) as a fixed factor and DYAD as a random factor was used. For the comparison of FTO values between groups for only the beginning of the dialogue (i.e. all transitions up to detection of the first Mismatch), the Bayesian model shows a mean δ of -322 (milliseconds) with a 95% CI of [-462, -138] and a posterior probability $P(\delta > 0) = 1$. The model therefore provides unambiguous evidence for the observation that autistic dyads produced considerably longer silent gaps between turn transitions than non-autistic dyads in the early stages of dialogue. For the remainder of the dialogue, mean δ is -45 (milliseconds) with a 95% CI of [-150, 60] and a posterior probability $P(\delta > 0) = 0.77$. The low posterior probability and the 95% CI including zero by a large margin strongly suggest that there was no difference between the turn-timing of autistic and non-autistic dyads in the later stages of dialogue.

In a three-way distinction of dialogue stages, we can then focus on turn transitions which take place during discussion of the first Mismatch. The relevant model (with the three-way distinction BEFORE/DURING/AFTER DISCUSSION OF THE FIRST MISMATCH, otherwise identical to the model described directly above) shows that there is no robust group difference for this epoch, expressed through a mean δ of -98 with a 95% CI [-228, 31] and a posterior probability $P(\delta > 0) = 0.9$. While this indicates a clear trend towards shorter FTO values in non-autistic dyads (in line with the overall trend) during discussion of the first Mismatch, the inclusion of zero in the 95% CI and the relatively low posterior probability suggest that this is not a reliable difference between groups.

4.4.2 Categorical analysis of turn transitions

For another perspective on turn-timing results, the continuous FTO results as presented above were divided into five different classes. Any gaps or overlaps with an absolute duration of less than 100 ms were categorised as *smooth transitions.* Gaps or overlaps with an absolute duration of or exceeding 700 ms were categorised as *long gaps/overlaps* and the remaining transitions with an absolute duration of 100–699 ms were categorised as *short gaps/overlaps.*

The cut-off point at 700 ms was inferred from previous work showing that gaps of 700 ms or longer are perceived as unusual by listeners. This judgement seems to stand in a causal relationship with the corresponding listener expectation that long gaps of this kind will be followed by repair initiations or non-affiliating responses (such as negative answers to yes-no questions), an expectation borne out by production data (Kendrick 2015, Kendrick & Torreira 2015, Roberts & Francis 2013, Schegloff et al. 1977).

In the following, I will discuss results from this categorical perspective in detail in those cases where it is informative beyond what we have already learned from considering FTO values in a continuous analysis (in §4.4.1).

Considering the dialogue as a whole, the most obvious finding remains that there is no clear difference between groups; see Figure 4.8. Both groups have very similar proportions of *smooth* transitions (such with absolute FTO values under 100 ms; ASD: 17%, CTR: 18.5%). The most relevant finding may be that the ASD group produced a slightly higher proportion of unusually long gaps (≥700 ms; ASD: 17.8%, CTR: 14.1%). This difference is not very large, but as discussed above, listeners are very sensitive to unusually long transitions, and so pattern may nevertheless be perceived as noteworthy by conversational partners (or outside observers) and therefore contribute to overall subjective impressions of diverging conversational behaviour.

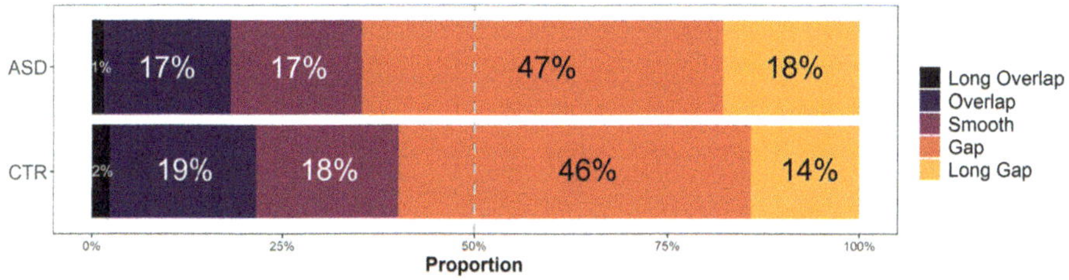

Figure 4.8: Stacked bar charts by group showing proportions of different transition types. ASD group on top, CTR group below. Transition proportions on the x-axis: long overlap transitions (FTO ≤ -700 ms) in black, overlaps (FTO -699 ms – -100 ms) in dark purple, very short (*smooth*) transitions (FTO -99 – 99 ms) in light purple, gaps (FTO 100 ms – 699 ms) in orange and long gaps (FTO ≥ 700 ms) in yellow.

A dyad-specific analysis shows that the group-level analysis accurately represents the behaviour of all dyads. The finding that there was a trend towards more long gaps in the ASD group is supported by the observation that four out of the five dyads with the highest long-gap proportions were autistic dyads, all with at least 19% long gaps – although the dyad with the single highest long-gap proportion was a CTR dyad (M11_M12, with 28.8% long gaps). Conversely, autistic dyads produced the three lowest proportions of long overlaps. It is also interesting to note that four out of the five lowest smooth transition proportions were produced by autistic dyads. Figure B.2 in Appendix B shows bar charts for all dyads.

Considering different stages of dialogue from a categorical perspective further corroborates results from the continuous FTO analysis: autistic dyads clearly differed in their turn-timing from control dyads only in the earliest stages of dialogue, after which they achieved a rhythm of turn exchanges equivalent to that of the CTR group. This can be visualised most vividly by only showing the proportions of long-gap transitions (≥700 ms FTO); see Figure 4.9. In the beginning of the dialogue (before detection of the first Mismatch), the proportion of long-gap transitions was more than twice as high for ASD dyads (29.1%) compared to CTR dyads (11.9%), but for the remaining dialogue there was practically no difference between groups (ASD: 16.8%; CTR: 14.4%). Not shown in Figure 4.9 is the fact that the reduction of long-gap transitions in the ASD group over time is mirrored by an increase for the same group in the proportion of smooth transitions (such with absolute values < 100 ms), with an increase from 11% to 18%.

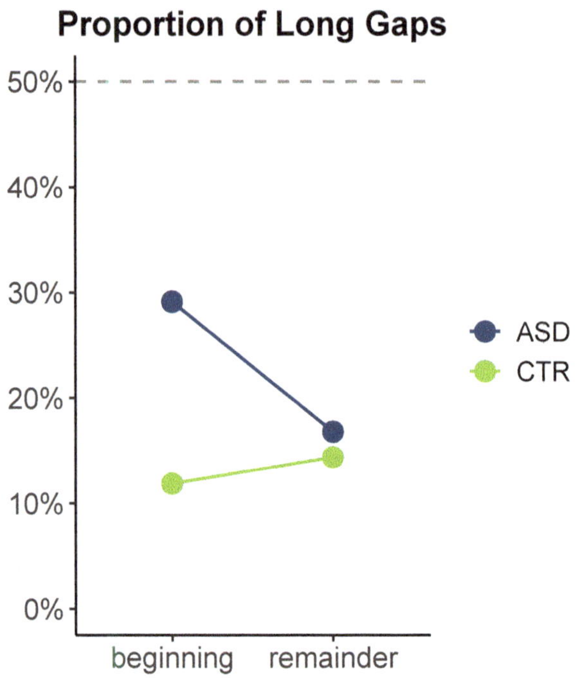

Figure 4.9: Proportions of long gap transitions (FTO ≥ 700 ms) by group and dialogue stage. Early stage of dialogue (before detection of first Mismatch) on the left, later stages of dialogue on the right. ASD group in blue, CTR group in green. Note that the y-axis is truncated at 50%.

4.4.3 Effects of unexpectedness: Matching and mismatching landmarks

In the preceding sections, different parts of dialogue were analysed by comparing the earliest stages – up to the first Mismatch – with the remainder of conversations. In this section, we will take a closer look at a subset of the data in only considering transitions directly following the introduction of new landmarks. The main interest here lies in comparing the effects of mismatching vs. matching landmarks. Mismatches are conceived of as a proxy for any unexpected events in social interaction, which many autistic speakers are said to struggle with.

To my knowledge, no other line of work has addressed the question of how matching vs. mismatching landmarks in the Map Task paradigm affect turn-taking behaviour (in any group of subjects).

4.4.3.1 Context, predictions and limitations

As participants in a Map Task cannot in any way be assumed to expect discrepancies between the two interlocutors' maps, mismatching landmarks should force participants to interrupt and discard their existing planning and adapt to unforeseen circumstances. Difficulties in dealing with situations involving change or unpredictable events are a typical clinical characteristic of ASD (American Psychiatric Association 2013: p. 50, Criterion B2). Recent phenomenological research on the subjective experience of time has corroborated that some autistic individuals not only evince reduced flexibility in planning, but also report a fear of unexpected events and interruptions in pre-planned time (Vogel et al. 2019).

As Mismatches are unexpected and atypical events within the task-oriented dialogue elicited through Map Tasks, we can hypothesise that they will cue repair initiations or similar responses. As discussed above, such responses have been associated with preceding extended gap transitions between speakers (≥700 ms). Therefore, gaps are predicted to generally be longer for Mismatches than for Matches.

Regarding the difference between Matches and Mismatches across groups, two alternative predictions can be considered:

1) It could be the case that turn-transitions differ more between Matches and Mismatches for the ASD as compared to the CTR group. This prediction follows the argument that individuals on the autism spectrum might be generally more sensitive to disturbances from unexpected events and might therefore also be affected more strongly by such events in the form of mismatching landmarks.

2) Alternatively, it could be the case that turn-transitions differ less between Matches and Mismatches for the ASD group compared to the control group. This prediction follows the argument that all new information, even in the form of expectable, matching landmarks, might be experienced as a kind of interruption for individuals on the autism spectrum, thus potentially levelling the playing field in the sense that Mismatches do not constitute a marked departure from difficulties that are already routinely experienced in conversation.

Although we are particularly interested in the effects of Mismatches as compared to Matches, the very nature of the Map Task means that there will always be considerably less data available for Mismatches. Not only is the effect of unexpectedness greatly reduced with each subsequent occurrence of a Mismatch, as will be seen, but the task would also be increasingly difficult to complete with the addition of more Mismatches – and some dyads struggle to complete the task with only the classic set-up involving two Mismatches. Therefore, an increase in mismatching landmarks would make breakdowns in conversation far more likely, yielding conversational data less representative of natural spoken interaction.

For these reasons, it is not feasible to analyse equal amounts of data for Matches and Mismatches. This might partly explain why there is no previous work investigating the effects of Mismatches on dialogue management in Map Tasks. As such, it is worth keeping in mind that this analysis might best be conceptualised as a qualitative case study. For the same reasons, i.e. paucity of (comparable) data, I will limit myself in this section to a purely descriptive account and forego Bayesian analysis as performed in other sections. Effect size estimation using Cohen's *d* (Cohen 1988) will be reported for the main results in order to give a clearer idea of differences between groups and types of landmark.

4.4.3.2 Data

All turn transitions following utterances in which a new landmark was introduced entered into analysis, except in the rare cases where more than one landmark was introduced within the same interpausal unit. In such cases, only the landmark that was mentioned last, at the end of the respective utterance, was included.

As this analysis is focussed on effects of unexpectedness, I will concentrate mainly on the first out of the two Map Tasks that each dyad completed. It will in fact be shown that effects of unexpectedness are already drastically diminished once the very first Mismatch (on the first set of maps) has been introduced.

The total number of turn transitions produced following the introduction of landmarks was 166 (123 after Matches, 43 after Mismatches). Note again the limited amount of data and, as a result, the inescapably qualitative character of this part of the analysis.

4.4.3.3 Results

I will first present a continuous and categorical analysis of turn-timing and then specifically consider 1) differences between the first and subsequent mismatching landmarks in the task as well as 2) differences between the first and the second Map Task.

Continuous analysis

A continuous FTO analysis shows that the CTR and the ASD group produced very similar turn-timing following Mismatches, in the form of long gaps around 700 ms. Note that this is a considerably higher mean FTO value than we have seen in the overall results (§4.4.1.1). Following Matches, however, the groups showed divergent behaviour, with the ASD group producing longer FTO values overall than the CTR group.

CTR speakers evinced turn-timing following Matches representative of typical values, as documented in the preceding sections and in previous studies. The mean FTO value for turn transitions after introduction of Matches in the CTR group was 101 ms (SD = 490). The respective density curve for the CTR data (grey curve in the right panel of Figure 4.10) shows a leptokurtic distribution with few extreme values and slightly more gaps than overlaps in the overall distribution.

ASD speakers on the other hand produced an unusually high mean FTO value of 433 ms (SD = 863) in transitions following the introduction of Matches. Although the median FTO value and the overall shape are similar to that of the CTR group, we can see a platykurtic distribution skewed towards the right, indicating more and longer gaps, which account for the difference in mean values (grey curve in the left panel of Figure 4.10). A comparison of FTO values following Matches between groups using Cohen's *d* reveals an effect size of 0.51 (medium effect size) (Cohen 1988, Sawilowsky 2009).

Following the introduction of Mismatches, the ASD and the CTR group behaved in a strikingly similar way, producing median FTO values of approximately 700 ms (ASD: 745ms; CTR: 724ms) and means of around 900 ms (ASD: 920 ms (SD = 805); CTR: 857 ms (SD = 744); see yellow density curves in Figure 4.10). These FTO values represent long gaps, such as typically occur in situations involving repair initiations due to misunderstanding or disagreement.

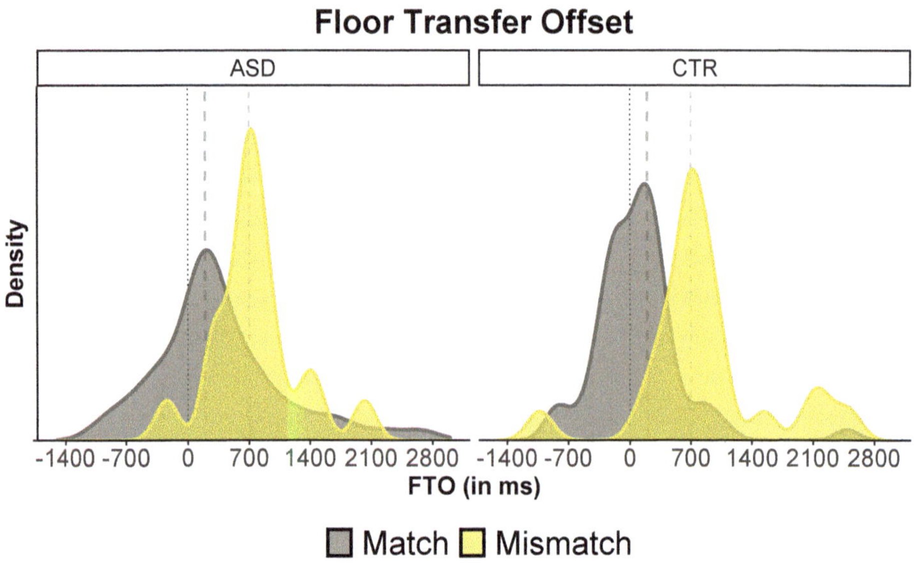

Figure 4.10: Density plot of FTO values in milliseconds, by group and Match/Mismatch. Negative values represent overlaps; positive values represent gaps. ASD group on the left, control group on the right. FTO values on the x-axis, density on the y-axis. FTO values for matching landmarks are represented in grey; FTO values for mismatching landmarks are presented in yellow.

Therefore, differences in turn transitions between the two groups were negligible where mismatching landmarks occurred. A comparison of FTO values following Mismatches between groups using Cohen's *d* reveals an effect size of 0.08 (negligible effect size).

Within groups, FTO values differed more between Matches and Mismatches for the CTR group (Cohen's d = 1.36; large effect size) than for the ASD group (Cohen's d = 0.58; medium effect size), as represented by the degree of overlap between the grey and yellow curves in Figure 4.10. In other words, there was a difference in turn-timing following Matches and Mismatches for both groups, but this difference was less pronounced in the ASD compared to the CTR group.

Analyses at the dyad-level largely confirm these patterns, although there was a very high degree of variability in the ASD group.

Categorical analysis

A categorical perspective can be particularly useful for the specific case of matching vs. mismatching landmarks. Here, the same categorisation of transition types as in §4.4.2 is used – dividing into long overlaps, overlaps, smooth transitions, gaps and long gaps – but, importantly, a *No Response* category is added.

As the name suggests, this category is used whenever a new landmark was introduced in the Map Task by the instruction giver, but not verbally acknowledged by the instruction follower. In other words, no floor transfer took place (and no response token was produced). These cases are treated (and visualised) as being conceptually adjacent to (very) long gaps. In essence, silence in such cases was simply maintained by the instruction follower for such a long time (1711 ms on average in the current data set) that the instruction giver eventually felt entitled (or obliged) to self-select for the next turn, thereby precluding any kind of turn transition between speakers. The expected silent gap between speakers following a turn-relevance place was in these cases effectively replaced with a period of intra-speaker silence (cf. Sacks et al. 1974).

Although the following results are presented as proportions of all transitions, it is important to keep in mind the very limited sample size for this subset of the data (absolute numbers are reported to add a sense of scale and context).

As can be seen in Figure 4.11, No Response cases (represented in beige) were less common in the CTR group. In fact, there is only one such instance following the introduction of matching landmarks (1.4%), and none at all following the introduction of mismatching landmarks. In the ASD group, fewer instances of newly introduced landmarks were verbally acknowledged. There were six cases of non-response following Matches (9.8%) and, strikingly, two instances following Mismatches (8.7%) as well.

Concerning the remaining transition types, we can see that following Matches (Panel A in Figure 4.11), ASD dyads produced more long gaps (32.8%; n = 20) than CTR dyads (7.2%; n = 5). Conversely, ASD dyads produced fewer overlaps and smooth (very short) transitions than control dyads. These differences were much less evident following Mismatches (Panel B in Figure 4.11), with both groups producing a similarly large proportion of long gaps, very few overlaps and no smooth (very short) transitions whatsoever.

Comparison of first vs. second Mismatch and Map Task

To further test the assumption that unexpectedness played a role in these results, we can compare transition times following utterances introducing the first vs. the second Mismatch within a map as well as in the first vs. in the second Map Task within a dialogue.

First, transitions following the first and the second Mismatch within the first Map Task will be compared. Although the distributions for both the ASD and the

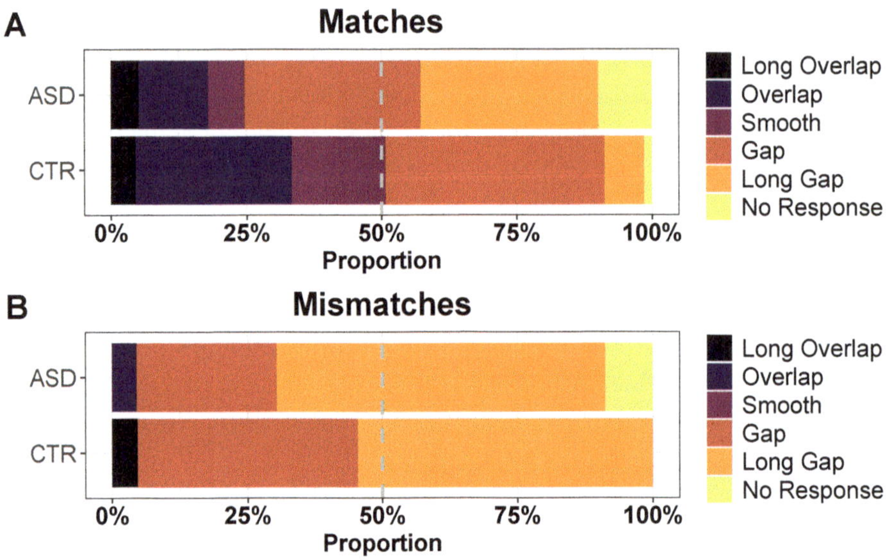

Figure 4.11: Stacked bar charts by group showing proportions of different types of turn transition. Values for matching landmarks in panel A (top), values for mismatching landmarks in panel B (bottom). Both panels contain two bars, with proportions for ASD participants on top and proportions for CTR participants below. Transition proportions on the x-axis: long overlap transitions (FTO ≤ -700 ms) in black, overlaps (FTO -699 ms – -100 ms) in dark purple, very short (*smooth*) transitions (FTO -99 – 99ms) in light purple, gaps (FTO 100 ms – 699 ms) in red, long gaps (FTO ≥ 700 ms) in orange and non-responses (no verbal reaction to mention of landmark) in beige.

CTR group peak at around 700 ms following mentions of either the first or the second Mismatch, the distributions for the first Mismatch are more variable and skewed considerably towards longer gaps (reflected in an across-groups mean value of 1228 ms; values were nearly identical across groups) compared with the second Mismatch (mean = 887 ms), as shown in Figure 4.12. This analysis also makes it clear that there were virtually no overlapping transitions after the introduction of Mismatches (in Map 1). These results seems to confirm the assumption that effects of unexpectedness will be diminished with the introduction of subsequent Mismatches.

Zooming out and considering differences between the first and the second Map Task within a recorded dialogue, we can see that, following completion of the first task, the effects associated with unexpectedness diminished. In other words, transitions following Mismatches had shorter FTO values in Map 2 compared to

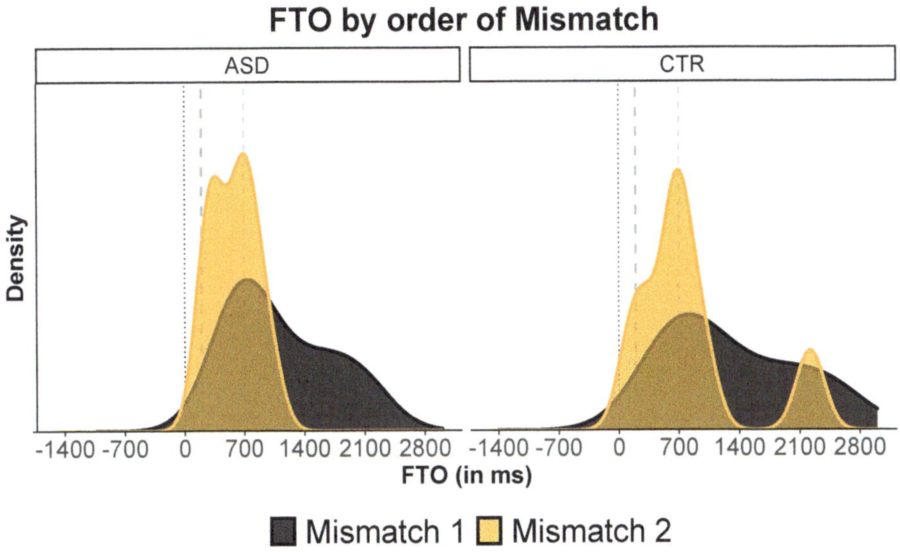

Figure 4.12: Density plots of FTO values by group and order of Mismatch. First Mismatch in the dialogue in black, second Mismatch in orange. ASD group on the left, CTR group on the right.

Map 1 overall, with some interesting group differences.

For the ASD group, FTO values in Map 2 were similar following Matches (mean = 350 ms; SD = 586) and Mismatches (mean = 480 ms; SD = 630). The effect size of this difference is small (Cohen's *d* = 0.21), smaller still than for the same comparison in Map 1 (*d* = 0.58; see §4.4.3.3).

For the CTR group, there was a greater difference than in the ASD group between FTO values following Matches (mean = 273 ms; SD = 304) and Mismatches (mean = 622 ms; SD = 605) in Map 2 (as for Map 1). The effect size of this difference is medium (Cohen's *d* = 0.74). This difference is greater than for the same comparison within the ASD group, but still far smaller than for the same comparison within the CTR group in Map 1 (*d* = 1.36; see §4.4.3.3).

In sum, turn transitions following Mismatches were shorter in Map 2 compared to Map 1, likely reflecting a diminished effect of unexpectedness and a concordant decrease in misunderstandings and the need for repair.

In the next section, we will expand our focus once again and consider the entire data set in concentrating on aspects beyond turn transitions.

4.4.4 Beyond transitions: Within-overlaps, signal analysis and speaking times

In this section, I will first present an analysis of within-speaker overlaps (where no floor transfer to another speaker takes place), including the presence or absence of backchannels in overlap. Second, overall proportions of silence (i.e. within-speaker pauses combined with between-speaker gaps) compared to overlapping and single-speaker speech will be considered, including an analysis of the distribution of overall speaking times within dyads.

4.4.4.1 Within-speaker overlaps

Within-overlaps are cases where a portion of overlapping speech is not followed by the floor being transferred to another speaker (in direct contrast to between-overlaps, as laid out in §4.3 and Figure 4.1). I will briefly characterise the nature and distribution of within-overlaps across groups in this section. In short, and similarly to overall turn-timing behaviour, results were comparable for autistic and non-autistic dyads.

Within-overlaps were typically very short, with an almost identical average duration across groups. The mean within-overlap duration for the ASD group was 380 ms (SD = 290) and the median was 314 ms. The mean within-overlap duration for the control group was 382 ms (SD = 279) and the median was 300 ms.

Not coincidentally, these durations almost exactly equal the mean duration of backchannels in the data set (378 ms; SD = 158), as 71.6% of ASD within-overlaps and 70% of CTR within-overlaps contained backchannels (and often consisted solely of a single backchannel). Overlaps containing backchannels can be considered *principled* or *sanctioned.* In other words, such overlaps don't constitute true interruptions, as backchannels are listener signals encouraging the interlocutor to hold the floor, rather than being the start of a competing turn by the interlocutor (see Chapter 5 for an in-depth analysis of backchannelling behaviour). Conversely, then, 28.4% of ASD within-overlaps and 30% of CTR within-overlaps can be considered true interruptions, of a kind that was not resolved by a floor transfer.

Although the group-level pattern reflects the behaviour of individual dyads accurately overall, it is interesting to note that the three dyads with the largest proportions of unprincipled overlaps (i.e. not containing backchannels) were dyads from the ASD group (≥60% unprincipled overlaps in each case).

Around 50% of *between-overlaps*, which were part of the FTO analyses in the preceding sections, also contained, or consisted solely of, one or multiple backchannels (ASD: 53.1%; CTR: 52.1%). It was ascertained that excluding these backchannel-containing overlaps does not change the results from the FTO analysis in any meaningful way, and therefore overlaps containing backchannels were included in the analysis of turn transitions reported above.

4.4.4.2 Overall signal: Silence, overlap and single-speaker speech

In the following, all IPUs and the silent spaces between them are considered (and not only turn transitions, as in the preceding sections).

Both groups of speakers produced virtually identical proportions of silence, overlaps and single-speaker speech. In both cases, almost three quarters of dialogue were taken up by speech from a single speaker (ASD: 72.5%; CTR: 73.1%), almost one quarter consisted of silence within or between speakers (ASD: 24%; CTR: 22.2%) and the small remainder was made up of overlapping speech from both interlocutors (ASD: 3.5%; CTR: 4.7%).

These results are remarkable for their great consistency not only across groups, but also across dyads (as shown in Figure B.3 in Appendix B). This finding adds to the extensive evidence in favour of the assertion made (prior to availability of any extensive quantitative evidence) in Sacks et al. (1974) that "[i]t has become obvious that, overwhelmingly, one party talks at a time" (p. 699).

Considering the overall amount of speech material, we can observe that speakers from the CTR group produced almost exactly twice as many IPUs (12121) as those from the ASD group (6211). This is mainly, but not entirely, due to the fact that ASD dyads were on average considerably quicker to complete the Map Tasks (mean time to completion: 14 minutes 40 seconds) than CTR dyads (mean: 26 minutes). Dialogue durations ranged from 9 minutes (ASD dyad M04_M05) to 49 minutes (CTR dyad M09_M10). Dyads from the ASD group accounted for the four shortest dialogues, while dyads from the CTR group accounted for four out of the five longest dialogues.

Although average dialogue durations were subject to a high degree of by-dyad variability in both groups, Bayesian modelling confirms a robust difference between groups. Linear regression with a log-normal distribution was used for the measure of overall dialogue duration in seconds ($\delta = 566$; 95% CI [51, 1149]; $P(\delta > 0) = 0.97$; details in the accompanying files).

The other main reason why there are more IPUs in the CTR group (in total and per minute of dialogue) is that in CTR dialogues, dyads produced more turn transitions. In other words, dialogues between non-autistic individuals entailed more frequent switches between the roles of listener and speaker (i.e. floor transfers per minute of dialogue).

Correspondingly, CTR dyads produced shorter utterances overall. IPUs produced by one speaker at a time (as opposed to speech from both interlocutors at once) had a mean duration of 1318 ms (SD = 1277) in the CTR group and 1424 ms (SD = 1369) in the ASD group (note the high degree of variability). Furthermore, portions of overlapping speech tended to be longer in the CTR group, but silences tended to be longer in the ASD group. Effect sizes are very small in both cases, however, and are unlikely to indicate any truly meaningful or generalisable differences.

Taking speaker roles (instruction giver/follower) into account allows us to observe that, rather unsurprisingly, instruction givers had about twice as much speaking time (52.1%) as instruction followers (24.1%) on average. This pattern is consistent across groups as well as dyads and can, to some extent, be explained by the fact that IPUs were longer for instruction givers (mean = 1526 ms; SD = 1366) than for instruction followers (mean = 1089 ms; SD = 1170).

4.4.4.3 Speaking time within dyads

In this section, I will introduce a measure for relative speaking times within dyads. This score simply indicates whether and to what extent one speaker within a dyad spoke more than the other. For instance, if 70% of a dialogue consists of single-speaker speech, in a perfectly balanced dyad speech from each interlocutor would account for one half of that (or 35% of the total), resulting in a score of 0. In other words, in such a perfectly balanced dyad, speech from each of the two participants would have the same overall duration. The lower the score, the more balanced the contributions from the two interlocutors. That is, if one person spoke more than the other, say with speech by Speaker A taking up 30% of overall dialogue duration and speech by Speaker B taking up 40% of overall duration, the resulting score would be 10 (40 - 30).

As can be seen in Figure 4.13, there was a clear tendency for autistic dyads to be less well-balanced in terms of speaking time. In the CTR group, four out of seven CTR dyads had almost perfectly equal speaking times (less than 1% difference in overall speaking time for the lowest three), whereas in the ASD group, only one out of seven dyads had a score of less than 5. In line with the other analyses presented in this work, this pattern does, however, not signify that there was a clear line that could be drawn between the behaviour of the two groups, due to pervasive dyad-specific effects. For instance, one ASD dyad had very balanced speaking times and one CTR dyad was one of the least balanced overall. The average score across groups was 10 for the ASD group and 5 for the CTR group.

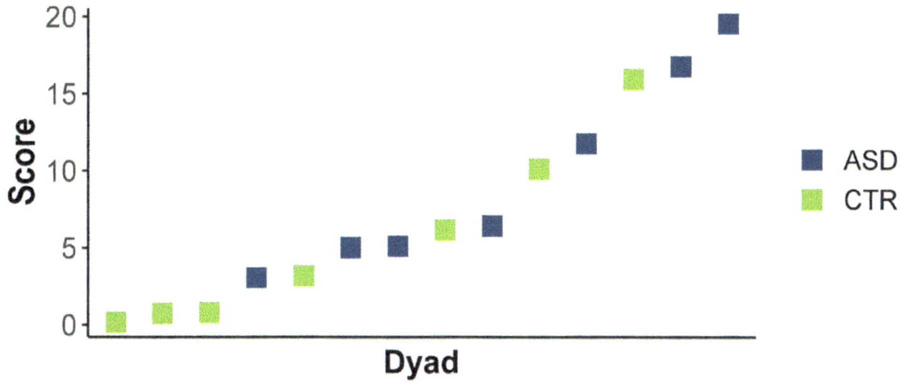

Figure 4.13: Speaking times within dyads. The lower the score, the more balanced the speaking times of the interlocutors within one dyad. ASD group in blue, CTR group in green.

As mentioned above, instruction givers tended to have twice as much speaking time as instruction followers. Combined with the fact that, for many dyads, Map Task 2 took less time to complete than Map Task 1, it follows that one speaker was instruction giver for longer than the other in such dyads. A detailed qualitative investigation confirms that this played no important role in accounting for overall speaking times, however, as dialogue in the later stages of longer Map Tasks consisted of relatively balanced input from both speakers in most cases.

4.4.4.4 Overview plots

Finally, I will present visualisations of the conversational data underlying all the different findings discussed in this book, such as turn-timing and speaker contributions, but also length of task and further aspects discussed in later chapters such as backchannels and filled pauses, in one single plot per dyad.

A *Praat* script was used to separately plot all IPUs for both speakers within each dyad, with special annotations for backchannels and filled pauses and highlighting time frames for detection, discussion and resolution of the first Mismatch. The script was adapted from the method used and discussed in Sbranna, Cangemi, et al. (2021), which in turn has many commonalities with the visualisation techniques used in Trouvain & Truong (2013), Campbell (2007); see Cangemi et al. (2023) for a further application and extension of this approach in the context of schizophrenia.

I will present and briefly describe two example plots below. The rest of the plots can be found in the folder "turnation" of the accompanying repository at https://osf.io/6vynj/ (for in-depth inspection, it is ideal to view these plots on screen as individual files).

Plots can be read like the written page in the Western tradition, i.e. from left to right and top to bottom. Each horizontal line represents one minute. Interpausal units are represented as red and blue lines (one colour per speaker). Backchannels are marked with lighter colours (pink and cyan, respectively). Filled pauses are marked in grey. The section of the dialogue from detection to resolution of the first Mismatch is marked with a green dotted line. The white space in the middle of each dialogue shows the time between completion of Map Task 1 and start of Map Task 2 (these data did not enter into analysis).

It is rather straightforward in this depiction to identify speaker roles, types of turn transition, frequency and timing of backchannels and filled pauses as well as overall task duration and different stages of dialogue. Most quantitative results can be directly related to the overview plots in this way.

Our first example is dyad F23_M22, from the control group. The overview plot is shown in Figure 4.14. This dyad was chosen as it is representative of the average behaviour in the CTR group in many regards. Map Task 1 and Map Task 2 were completed within 16 minutes, with about 8 minutes spent on each task – shorter than average for the CTR group. In both cases, the instruction giver (red in Map 1; blue in Map 2) has far more speaking time than the follower. Overall, however, speaking times were almost perfectly balanced, with a difference score of only 0.2 (percent proportional to overall dialogue duration). The first Mismatch was detected quickly and resolved in a relatively short amount of time. There were slightly more floor transfers per minute than average, resulting also in a slightly shorter average IPU length. The mean FTO for turn-timing was 220 ms, typical for this group of speakers as well as for results from previous studies. The rates of backchannels (pink/cyan), filled pauses (grey) and silent pauses (white spaces within turns) produced were very close to the group average.

Our second example is dyad M07_M08, from the ASD group. The overview plot is shown in Figure 4.15. This dyad was chosen as it represents relatively unusual behaviour along several dimensions. Here, overall task duration was very short, with a total of only 10 minutes. Speaker M07 (blue lines) has considerably more speaking time than speaker M08 overall, taking many turns in the roles of both instructor (Map 1) and follower (Map 2). Overall, M07_M08 was the second least well-balanced dyad in terms of speaking time within a dyad, with a score of

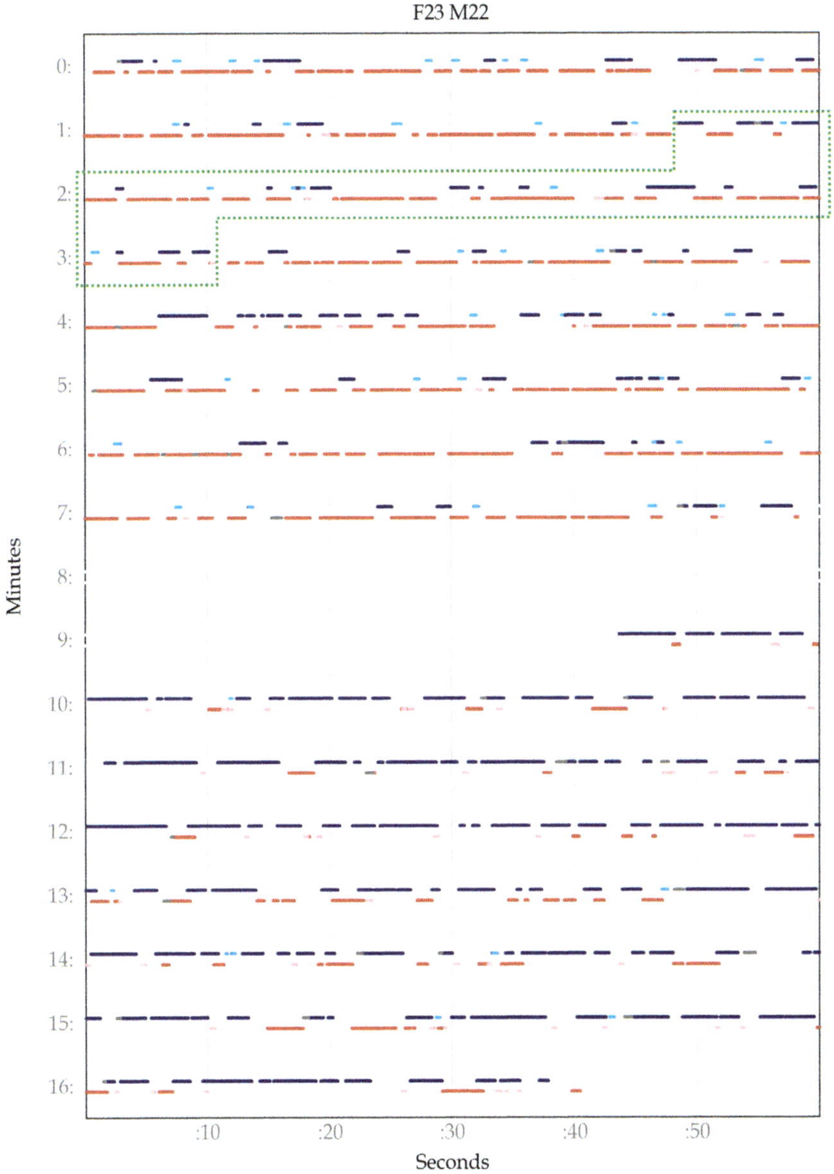

Figure 4.14: Overview plot for dyad F23_M22 from the CTR group. Speaker F23 in blue, speaker M22 in red. Backchannels in lighter colours (pink/cyan), filled pauses in grey. The section of dialogue from detection to full resolution of the first Mismatch is outlined in green.

17. The dyad produced a relatively low number of floor transfers per minute, resulting in an unusually high mean IPU duration. The first Mismatch was detected quickly, but took a relatively long time to be resolved. Although FTO was close to the group average, the dyad produced an unusually high proportion of long gaps (≥700 ms). Dyad M07_M08 produced by far the lowest rate of backchannels per minute (pink/cyan) and a relatively high rate of both filled pauses (grey) and silent pauses (white spaces within turns).

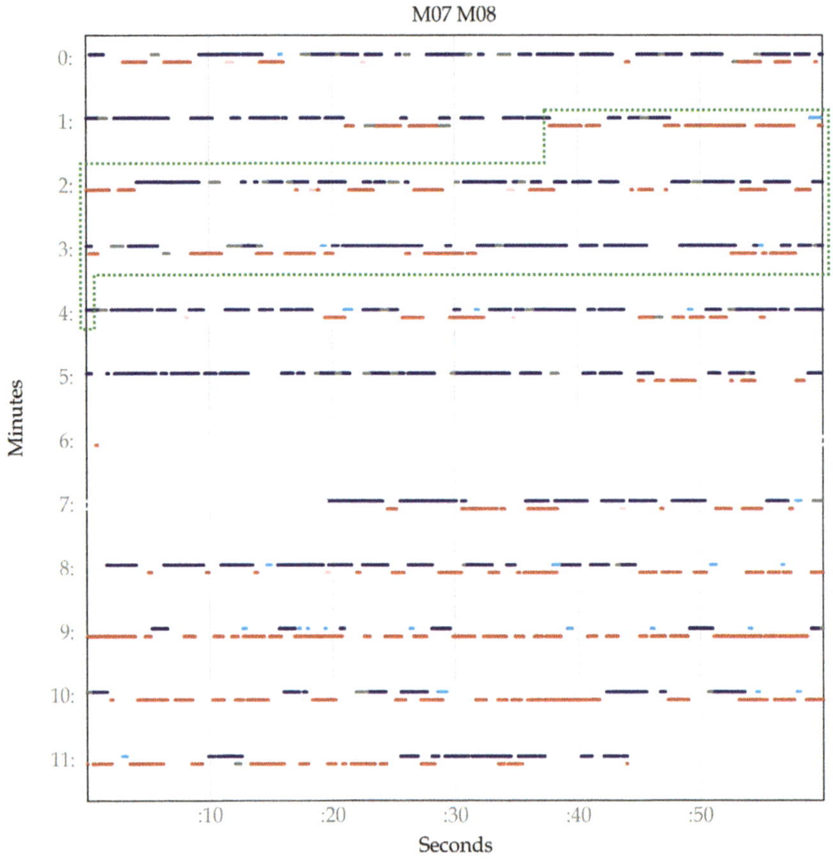

Figure 4.15: Overview plot for dyad M07_M08 from the ASD group. Speaker M07 in blue, speaker M08 in red. Backchannels in lighter colours (pink/cyan), filled pauses in grey. The section of dialogue from detection to full resolution of the first Mismatch is outlined in green.

I will refer back to some of the overview plots in the general discussion (Chapter 6), where findings from the different parts of this book are tied together in order to reveal general characteristics of conversation and intonation for each ASD dyad.

4.4.5 Prosodic realisation

Although the analysis of turn-timing in this book does not specifically focus on prosodic aspects, I did examine whether speakers used intonational cues to turn-ends (and beginnings) in ways that are comparable between groups and to what has been reported in previous studies. In this section, I will give a brief insight into methods and results, reserving a full account for future publications.

Examples for commonly found prosodic constructions are downstep, late pitch peak, or, more closely related to the current investigation, turn-switch and back-channelling. Dimensions are automatically extracted from a given data set along with summary plots and a list of time-stamped examples of the relevant construction. Identifying the significance and function of the dimensions provided by the automatic PCA procedure is left to the researcher. However, by inspecting the summary plots and relating them to the list of examples in the data set, as well as to previous research using the method, it is very straightforward to identify the most common constructions.

The most relevant construction for the investigation of turn-timing is what Ward (2019) calls the "Basic Turn-Switch Construction" (also discussed in Ward & Gallardo 2017). Ward (2019) describes this construction as follows:

> About a second before ending a turn, the speaker typically produces a bundle of characteristic features, including higher pitch, narrower pitch range, and lengthening. This is followed by a region of lower pitch and increased creakiness, and then a half second later the turn end....the prosody afterwards, as the new speaker takes the turn, is also significant. As the loadings suggest, this commonly is high in pitch, and also loud, reduced and creaky (pp. 142–145).

The results of PCA applied to the current data set reveal that both groups of speakers marked turn ends and beginnings in a way that is highly compatible with the above description. More importantly, there was no obvious difference between groups. None of this should come as too much of a surprise, given that 1) we have seen that all dyads in the data set under study produced typically rapid turn-timing for the vast majority of the dialogue and 2) experimental evidence suggests that such split-second precision in turn-timing is only possible when all relevant linguistic cues, including prosodic cues, are present in the signal (Barthel et al. 2017, 2016, Bögels & Levinson 2017, Bögels & Torreira 2015, Torreira & Bögels 2022).

Figure 4.16 shows the loadings of the relevant dimension in the PCA analysis for both the CTR and the ASD group. These plots closely resemble the example given in Ward (2019: p. 143). This confirms that the present findings, for both groups, are compatible with those of previous studies. Specifically, turn-endings in the data set under study tended to be marked by falling pitch, lengthening and creakiness, while turn-beginnings tended to be marked by high pitch, high intensity and creakiness.

The plots are read such that the top half of each graph represents one speaker in a dialogue and the bottom half represents their interlocutor. Time flows from left to right on the x-axis and plots are centred at the core of the prosodic construction at 0 milliseconds – in this case the precise moment of turn transition from one speaker to the next. For each parameter, as the relevant curve goes up beyond the central line, values are higher than average and as it goes down, values are lower than average. If we focus, for instance, on the line representing intensity, we can see that intensity drops (to silence) at the zero-millisecond mark for the speaker on top, while it rises (from silence) for the other speaker (in both the CTR and the ASD group).

These results clearly indicate that prosodic aspects of turn-taking were equivalent across groups and that the intonational marking of turn ends and beginnings conforms to what has been reported in previous studies. One shortcoming of the PCA approach is that it is not very well suited to in-depth analysis at the dyad level, or of shorter time windows (e.g. for an analysis of the earliest stages of dialogue only). Not enough data are available in such cases to guarantee a robust analysis with reliable extraction of all relevant dimensions. Thus, it remains for future studies to investigate prosodic aspects of dyad-specific behaviour as well as differences between different stages of dialogue. From a more general perspective, the approach demonstrated here might be used to narrow the still considerable gap between quantitative and qualitative traditions in research on turn-taking (and conversation analysis more generally). Such an approach is already inherent in the methodology designed and described by Ward (2019), as the decidedly quantitative computational black box that is PCA is here employed to produce a list of timestamped examples of conversational behaviour which are then to be examined and described qualitatively and in great detail. In this way, the sheer analytical power of quantitative approaches can be harnessed in order to facilitate the detection of examples best suited to an in-depth qualitative analysis.

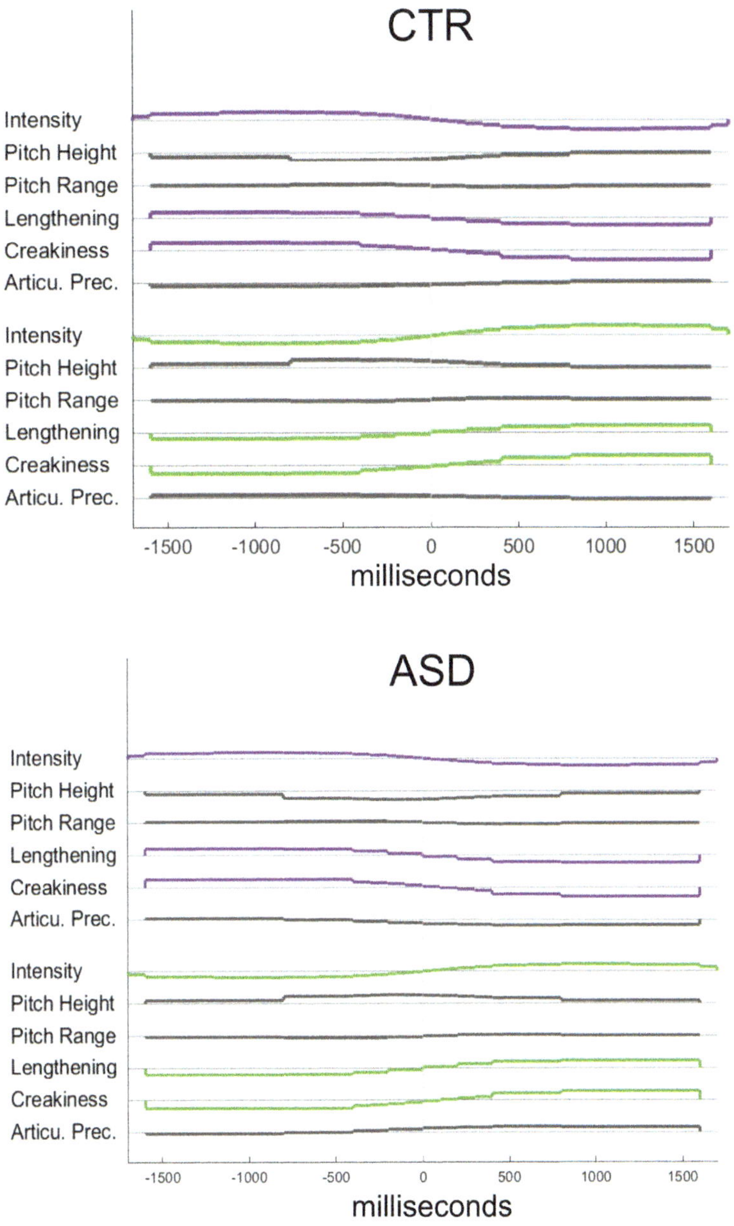

Figure 4.16: Loading plots for the Basic Turn-Switch Construction as revealed by principal component analysis. CTR group on top, ASD group on the bottom. See text for details.

4.5 Discussion

To conclude this chapter, I will summarise the relevant findings, discuss their implications, situate them in the landscape of previous research, point out the limitations of the study and sketch some directions for future work.

4.5.1 Summary

An in-depth analysis of turn-timing in German-speaking adults with and without a diagnosis of autism spectrum disorder was presented. This is the first study of turn-timing in conversations between autistic adults and one of the first in-depth studies of turn-timing in German. It was found that autistic dyads behaved similarly to non-autistic dyads in many respects. For example, there was no reliable group-difference for overall FTO values (representing the timing of turns). A closer look at different stages of dialogue revealed that autistic dyads did in fact behave differently from control dyads, but only in the earliest stages of dialogue, where they produced more long gaps.

Another difference between groups was found in the realisation of turn transitions directly following the introduction of new landmarks. Both groups reacted to mismatching landmarks early in the task by producing many long gaps, reflecting the fact that such unexpected events are almost bound to lead to misunderstanding and repair. However, only the ASD group produced a similarly high proportion of long gaps following the introduction of *matching* landmarks.

It is important to point out that turn-timing behaviour, as all other aspects of intonation and dialogue management discussed in this book, revealed no clear dividing line between the ASD group and the CTR group. Dyad-specific analyses have shown that around half of the autistic dyads showed behaviour within the range of CTR dyads for most of the dimensions investigated.

It was further shown that, for both groups, overlaps within speaker turns were typically very short, often consisting only of a single backchannel token, and that half of all overlaps contained backchannels. The speaking times between interlocutors within dyads tended to be less balanced in the ASD group. Finally, no group difference in the prosodic realisation of turn-ends and turn-beginnings was found.

4.5.2 Implications and interpretation

In the following, I will discuss the implications of some of the results covered in this chapter and place them in the context of previous research. I will first cover overall turn-timing and then the subset of transitions following the introduction of new landmarks, and conclude with a brief comparison of results on turn-taking in ASD with results on turn-taking in second language speech.

4.5.2.1 Turn-timing: Longer gaps in the early stages of conversation

The finding that differences in turn-taking between groups, in the form of longer gaps in the conversations of autistic dyads, were found only in the earliest stages of dialogue shows that autistic speaker pairs successfully established a degree of rapid turn-timing that is essentially indistinguishable from that of non-autistic dyads, but that they did not do so instantly (cf. Levitan et al. 2015). Arriving at such equivalent turn-timing behaviour appears to be literally a matter of time for dyads in the ASD group, as it seems to be independent of conversational content (here, progress in the Map Task or, more specifically, encountering and discussing the first Mismatch).

Given that listeners are very sensitive to even small differences in turn-timing (Kendrick & Torreira 2015) and form personality impressions about speakers extremely rapidly (McAleer et al. 2014), the overall turn-taking style of the ASD group may still be perceived as odd or unusual, at least by typically developed listeners. This holds true even though there was no robust difference between autistic and non-autistic dyads for most of the dialogue – precisely because the relevant differences are found during the earliest stages of conversation.

These specific differences should, however, not overshadow the general finding that, at a global level, no robust differences were found in conversations between autistic as opposed to non-autistic adults. This might be considered surprising given that 1) it has been shown at length in previous work that achieving rapid and precise turn-timing is highly challenging cognitively, as it can only be achieved if speakers are able to accurately predict the communicative intentions of their interlocutor (Bögels & Torreira 2015, De Ruiter et al. 2006, Gleitman et al. 2007, Wesseling & van Son 2005, Barthel et al. 2016), and 2) predicting the behaviour of others is a skill that many autistic individuals seem to struggle with (Cannon et al. 2021).

The current findings clearly show that at least the kinds of relatively socially motivated and skilled autistic adults investigated in this study, and at least when conversing in disposition-matched (ASD–ASD) dyads, are perfectly able to produce turn-timing of the same speed and precision as has been described for conversations between adults without a diagnosis of ASD. The related observations that, compared to the CTR group, speakers in the ASD group did not use more filled pauses (see §5.4) and produced turn-ends and beginnings with the same intonational realisation as the CTR group (see §4.4.5) furthermore discourage alternative explanations for equivalent turn-timing across the two groups (e.g. that although the utterances of autistic dyads were produced with the same timing, they may have differed in terms of informativeness or prosodic detail). An alternative or complementary theory would be that factors such as perspective-taking or Theory of Mind simply play less of a role in turn-taking (and perhaps even ASD in general; see Williams 2021) than has previously been assumed.

The results presented here extend the numerous findings on the apparent universality of turn-timing for the first time to conversations between autistic adults. On the one hand, this strengthens the notion that turn-taking is a fundamental aspect of human interaction, and one that is apparently very similar across groups of speakers with different cognitive, cultural and linguistic backgrounds. On the other hand, the subtle differences between the CTR group and the ASD group detected by taking into account temporal dynamics suggest that similarly subtle differences between other groups of speakers may yet to be discovered. It is possible that a focus on the undeniably remarkable similarities of turn-timing across populations and contexts has overshadowed subtle differences at smaller scales, which might only be discovered with the use of more fine-grained qualitative and quantitative approaches.

4.5.2.2 Transitions following expected vs. unexpected information

An analysis of only the turn transitions following the introduction of new landmarks revealed that both groups produced long gaps of around 700 milliseconds following the introduction of mismatching landmarks. This is a value typical of situations involving misunderstanding, non-affiliating answers or repair initiations, which featured prominently in almost all interactions following the introduction of at least the first landmark to unexpectedly differ between maps.

A difference between groups was found only for transitions following the introduction of *matching* landmarks. In these cases, no effects of misunderstanding or surprise are expected and indeed non-autistic dyads produced transitions with typical short gaps. Autistic dyads, on the other hand, produced longer gaps, meaning that in this group only, gaps were relatively long following the introduction of both *matching and mismatching* landmarks. Additionally, it was shown that ASD speakers in certain cases also provided no verbal reaction to the introduction of new landmarks, even for Mismatches.

It is highly unusual not to explicitly acknowledge new – albeit expected – information (see the 1.5% non-response rate following Matches for the control group). However, such verbal acknowledgement is not strictly necessary from a functional perspective. Cases such as the 10.9% of non-responses following Matches for the ASD group do not directly prevent participants from being able to complete the Map Task by transferring the given route from one map to the other. This is not true, however, in the case of Mismatches. Here, it would seem necessary to directly address the issue at hand and to initiate a repair, or question the interlocutor's statement, in order to re-establish or strengthen common ground and be in a position to complete the task appropriately. Hence, the 8.7% rate of non-responses in Mismatches for the ASD group is particularly striking, especially when considering that all 14 speakers in the control group addressed each single occurrence of a Mismatch explicitly and verbally (always keeping in mind the low sample size, which limits the generalisability of this finding).

The relatively frequent occurrence of long gaps and non-responses for both kinds of landmark suggests that autistic dyads treated new information, whether it was matching or mismatching across maps, as unexpected more often than control dyads, who only showed a high proportion of long gaps in response to unusual and unexpected events in the form of mismatching landmarks.

In principle, there could be many reasons for the longer between-turn gaps in the ASD group. General delays in response production have been attested for individuals on the autism spectrum in various studies on motor production, language production and language perception (see e.g. Gernsbacher et al. 2008). However, as the ASD group only differed from controls for Matches, and not for Mismatches, it seems necessary to provide more specific explanations for this difference. It could be speculated that autistic subjects simply did not describe landmarks as clearly as controls, but a cursory content analysis suggests that this is not the case. A more likely, if no less speculative, explanation may be found in relating the current results to characteristic features of subjective time experience in ASD (Zukauskas et al. 2009).

It has been claimed that for individuals on the autism spectrum, the present is often experienced as a sequence of small, non-overlapping units or events which are planned in advance (broadly in line with theories of Weak Central Coherence; Frith 2003, Happé et al. 2001). This can result in a fear of outside events interrupting an individual's self-imposed and pre-planned temporal structure (Vogel et al. 2019). When unexpected outside influences do interrupt the present, the experience of time can appear discontinued and lead to what Vogel and colleagues refer to as "interrupted time experience". Time as experienced by most non-autistic persons, on the other hand, seems to more closely resemble a series of stretched-out and overlapping time windows with fuzzy boundaries (Vogel et al. 2020). This latter representation should be far more robust to interruptions and unexpected events (for instance in the shape of new information being conveyed by an interlocutor) than the string of discrete, sequential and non-overlapping units that has been described to characterise time perception for at least some autistic persons.

Applying this perspective to the current data, it could be speculated that subjective time experience in ASD was one reason for the fact that autistic dyads reacted to the introduction of all new information (expected or unexpected) by producing longer silent gaps – in contrast to non-autistic dyads, who produced longer gaps only directly following the unexpected introduction of *mismatching* landmarks, which inherently contain an element of surprise.

4.5.2.3 Comparison to turn-timing in non-native dialogues

As pointed out above, the turn-timing analysis presented in this work is directly comparable to only very few previously published studies. To expand the scope and provide a wider sense of context, the same analogy as in other parts of this book can be employed by comparing autistic language with bilingual, or non-native, language production.

Second language (L2) learners might be expected to produce more and longer silent gaps, as they are not only faced with the regular challenges inherent in performing rapid turn-timing, but additionally with the considerable and multi-faceted difficulties of communicating in a non-native language. This expectation is strengthened by the two adjacent findings that 1) word naming in L2 speech is delayed (Hanulová et al. 2011) and 2) the typical fast turn-timing patterns of adult conversation are not reached in *first* language acquisition until around the age of 9 (Casillas et al. 2016, Garvey & Berninger 1981).

To my knowledge, the first published study that includes a detailed discussion of results on turn-timing in non-native speech is Galaczi (2014). The author examined conversations between 41 dyads that were recorded as part of Cambridge English Language Assessment. Cambridge English is an exam board and organisation which made major contributions to the development of the European Union's Common European Framework of Reference for Languages (Council of Europe 2001) and continues to perform language assessments aligned with the proficiency levels set out in this framework. The work of Galaczi (2014) is conducted mostly in the tradition of qualitative Conversation Analysis. This entails an analysis of turn-timing which is rather coarse compared to the methods applied in this book. Specifically, only a categorical analysis with three distinct types of turn transitions was performed. Those categories were "latch/overlap" (corresponding to any negative FTO values), "no-gap-no-overlap" (any gaps of

500 milliseconds or less) and “pause” (gaps longer than 500 milliseconds). Describing gaps of 0 ms and 500 ms equally as “no-gap” is exemplary of the problematic simplifications inherent in this approach. Galaczi (2014) reports that L2 English speakers with a lower proficiency tended to produce slightly higher proportions of “pauses”, corresponding to longer silent intervals between speakers, than L2 speakers with higher proficiency levels.

A more recent study by Sørensen et al. (2019) tested native Danish speakers who were highly proficient in English performing a spot-the-difference task in both their L1 and their L2. The authors report that FTO values in L2 speech were either equivalent to those in L1 speech or, contrary to expectations, *lower* compared to L1 speech, depending on whether conversations took place in silence or in noise.

The results from these studies on non-native turn-timing can be related to the findings described in the current work and in previous studies on turn-taking in ASD. As the participants in the current study were motivated and socially skilled autistic adults, one could really only expect to see parallels (if any) with results from highly proficient L2 learners or bilingual speakers (as opposed to less advanced learners; cf. §6.2.7). Indeed, the current results and those on highly proficient L2 speakers in both Galaczi (2014) and Sørensen et al. (2019) reveal no differences in turn-timing compared to the relevant control groups (non-autistic native speakers). In contrast, results from previous work on autistic children more closely align with what was found for beginner learners of an L2 in Galaczi (2014) in revealing a tendency for longer silent gaps between speakers.

Although research on turn-taking in second-language speech is still very limited in scope, comparing non-native with autistic turn-timing holds promise for future investigations, especially since more in-depth analyses of L2 turn-timing have been proposed and exemplified recently in work by e.g. Sbranna, Cangemi, et al. (2021), Sbranna, Wehrle, et al. (2021).

4.5.3 Limitations, extensions and future directions

Although I believe that the thoroughness and transparency of the analysis allows us to draw certain conclusions on the basis of the experimental results with a certain degree of confidence, naturally there are many factors to limit external validity.

First, the behaviour of socially skilled German-speaking autistic adults was analysed. There are many ways in which results might differ for individuals situated at different points on the autism spectrum, of different native language backgrounds, and at different stages of development. The state of the art is such that we cannot directly compare the results at hand to any others on turn-timing in ASD. An obvious extension of the present work would therefore be replications with children and/or with adults speaking a language other than German.

Second, semi-spontaneous dialogues without eye contact between participants were elicited. A multi-modal analysis of video-recorded interactions between speakers with and without ASD could therefore add further crucial information, as gaze and gesture have been shown to play important roles in dialogue management (e.g. Mondada 2019, Auer 2018, McCleary & de Arantes Leite 2013, Holler et al. 2018, Zellers et al. 2016, Bohus & Horvitz 2010). Recent work by De Marchena et al. (2019) specifically shows that autistic speakers seemed to use gesture more than non-autistic speakers to regulate turn-timing. Follow-up experiments including recordings of gaze, posture and gesture are currently being conducted (Spaniol et al. 2023). Regarding the contextual constraints inherent in the Map Task, it is true that having to fulfil an unfamiliar task puts certain pressures and limitations on participants and the resulting linguistic output, and this may have affected speakers in the ASD group differently than those in the CTR group. However, the restricted set of dialogue options and reduced chance of unexpected events may in fact have suited the cognitive styles of autistic speakers more than fully free and spontaneous conversation, which would in turn make the between-group differences described in this paper all the more relevant.

Third, as the behaviour of disposition-matched dyads (ASD–ASD) was investigated here, perhaps most obvious would be an extension to also include mixed dyads (ASD–CTR). The overwhelming majority of experimental work on communication in ASD has in fact been conducted using mixed dyads only. Disposition-matched dyads (ASD–ASD) rather than mixed dyads (ASD–CTR) were recorded for two main reasons. First, there is quite simply a dramatic lack of research on communication in ASD based on data from such matched dyads. Second, investigating the behaviour of disposition-matched dyads seems to me the most promising way to gain insights into what might justifiably be called autistic communication. Analysing the behaviour of mixed dyads makes it very difficult to see beyond the patterns and potential difficulties arising from the interaction of individuals with different cognitive styles (Milton 2020, 2012, Williams et al. 2021, McCracken 2021). While such insights are of great value in principle, they cannot be interpreted conclusively and appropriately unless we first have a clear picture of what characterises communication between autistic speakers.

This perspective, in the sense of a certain epistemic humility, extends to the study at hand. For instance, while we can accurately say that the ASD group tended to produce longer silent gaps between turns than the CTR group in certain parts of conversations, by no means can (or should) we claim that this behaviour is simply "wrong" or "inappropriate" in any way. Not only do we have to recognise the very likely possibility that autistic dialogue strategies diverge from those of non-autistic peers in ways that are the most appropriate and functional for this group in the given situation. We also have to acknowledge that we cannot say for sure whether long gaps, produced by any group of speakers, are appropriate or not in a given context without conducting a comprehensive qualitative analysis that takes into account the context of turn transitions. Previous work assures us, for instance, that long gaps are typical and expected in the direct context of verbal exchanges involving misunderstanding or non-alignment (Kendrick & Torreira 2015, Kendrick 2015, Roberts & Francis 2013).

It is beyond the scope of this work to exhaustively analyse how many cases of long gaps were indeed produced in just such contexts for each group, but the detailed analysis of different stages of dialogue gives us a proxy for such an analysis. It was shown that gaps were longest for the ASD group before detection of the first Mismatch (whereas values were comparable throughout the dialogue for the CTR group). This makes it clear that these cases of long-gap transitions are not specifically linked to unexpected events as part of the task itself, but rather reflect the previously attested observation that people diagnosed with ASD tend to have more difficulties with, and tend to be less comfortable in, situations involving newness or uncertainty. Conversely, it was shown that dyads from the CTR and the ASD group produced equally long gaps immediately following the introduction of mismatching landmarks, but that dyads from the ASD group produced longer gaps immediately following the introduction of matching landmarks compared to the CTR group.

In essence, autistic dyads thus produced many long gaps in various situations sharing an element of novelty, while non-autistic dyads only produced long gaps in the context of particularly challenging aspects of the experimental task itself (such as the introduction of an unexpected mismatch). Generally speaking, using such long gaps may be an effective strategy for navigating challenging and unusual situations, and it is employed by both groups of speakers in the data set under study. The difference, then, lies only in the fact that this strategy was used by dyads from the ASD group in a wider variety of contexts. The best way to test such assertions experimentally would be to conduct perception tests in future studies. This would make it possible to assess and compare just how meaningful the differences in turn-timing found here are (perceived to be) for both autistic and non-autistic listeners, and to what extent such differences might influence understanding as well as character judgements.

I mentioned second-language speech as an analogous and similarly understudied area in research on turn-taking. This equally applies to communication in schizophrenia. Beyond a small number of published papers (Breitholtz et al. 2021, Howes et al. 2017, Lucarini et al. 2021, Cangemi et al. 2023), we do not know much about dialogue management in schizophrenia. A comparative study of turn-taking in ASD and in schizophrenia could help to shed light on differences and similarities between the two groups and, by extension, on social interaction and neurodiversity in general.

Finally, triadic instead of dyadic conversation, as investigated e.g. in the aforementioned studies by Auer (2018), Breitholtz et al. (2021) can serve as a highly promising extension to general findings on turn-taking in dialogue and could equally usefully be applied to the specific case of turn-taking in ASD.

5 Backchannels and filled pauses

5.1 Introduction

This part of the book is dedicated to a comparative analysis of backchannels (BC; listener signals such as *mmhm* or *okay*) and filled pauses (FP; hesitation signals such as *uhm*) by speakers with and without a diagnosis of autism spectrum disorder.

Backchannels are a ubiquitous and essential feature of spoken interaction. They are used predominantly by listeners to support the ongoing turn of the interlocutor and to signal understanding and agreement (see references in §5.3.1). Previous research has shown that listeners are highly sensitive to the exact realisations of backchannels and that they judge deviations from typical forms (by e.g. non-native speakers) as negative (e.g. Li 2006). Previous research on backchannelling in ASD is limited to two studies.

It was found that in the corpus of Map Task dialogues under investigation, the backchannel productions of autistic speakers were characterised by 1) a lower rate of BCs per minute (particularly in the early stages of dialogue), 2) less diversity in the use of different BC types and 3) a lower degree of flexibility and diversity in the mapping of different intonation contours to different BC types. These results can be interpreted as reflecting more general characteristics of autistic people engaged in communicative social interaction, namely differences in how and to what extent interest and attention are expressed towards an interlocutor as well as a tendency for more stable (or less flexible) patterns of behaviour.

Filled pauses are another kind of discourse marker which is extremely common in spontaneous speech (see references in §5.4.1). In contrast to backchannels, filled pauses are used by speakers to hold (or take) the floor (instead of giving up their own as of yet incomplete turn) and to signal hesitancy and inchoateness. Previous research on filled pauses in ASD is fairly limited and has yielded somewhat mixed results.

No differences between groups were found regarding the rate of filled pauses produced, nor the preference of one filled pause type (*uhm*) over the other (*uh*). In contrast, group differences were found for intonational realisation, with autistic speakers producing fewer FPs with the "default" level intonation contour and using a higher proportion of both falls and rises instead. Based on these results, claims from previous studies on the use of filled pauses in ASD are critically evaluated regarding the listener-oriented nature of filled pauses in general and of *uhm* in particular.

Finally, a number of related phenomena were examined, showing that 1) ASD dyads produced more long silent pauses, 2) there were longer silent intervals following *uhm* than following *uh* (independent of FP duration) in both groups and 3) CTR dyads produced more laughter per minute than ASD dyads.

Importantly, for all measures described in the rest of the chapter (and in the book as a whole), group differences were indicative of robust trends across speakers and dyads, but in all cases at least some autistic speakers and dyads behaved within the range of the CTR group. In other words, there was considerable overlap between the ASD and the CTR group.

In the following, I will first summarise the data and methods used and then turn to detailed analyses of backchannels and filled pauses. After a discussion of silent pauses and laughter, I will finally summarise and interpret the most important findings, point out limitations of the present study and suggest promising avenues for future investigations.

The backchannel analysis (§5.3) has previously been reported in Wehrle, Vogeley, et al. (2023a), the filled pause analysis (§5.4) in Wehrle, Grice & Vogeley (2023) and the silent pause analysis (§5.5) in Wehrle, Vogeley, et al. (2023b).

5.2 Data and analysis

The analysis is based on the same corpus of semi-structured Map Task dialogues referred to throughout the book (see Chapter 2), that is, on approximately 5 hours of speech produced by 28 native German adults, half of which had been diagnosed with autism spectrum disorder.

In total, 2371 backchannel tokens and 1027 filled pause tokens were extracted.

Backchannels were coded according to strict criteria, following the Acknowledgement move in Carletta et al. (1997), but excluding repetitions. Thereby, all utterances signalling that a speaker had heard and understood their interlocutor were initially included. Importantly, all of the following were then excluded: 1) turn-initial backchannels (where a backchannel directly precedes a more substantial utterance by the same speaker, e.g. "Okay, and what's next?"), 2) answers to polar questions (such as "Do you see this?") and 3) answers to tag questions (such as "Near the corner, right?"). The remaining utterances were, therefore, backchannels in a strict sense, as they were not part of a larger unit and were not explicitly invited by the interlocutor (e.g. through a question). Note that this operationalisation of backchannels differs markedly from looser categorisations such as the *VSU* (very short utterance) category used in e.g. Heldner et al. (2011), Sbranna et al. (2023); see Fujimoto (2009) for a discussion regarding issues of terminology in previous work on backchannels.

Filled pauses were defined as all hesitations roughly of the form 'äh' or 'ähm' in German. All tokens including a final nasal were included in the *uhm* category and all tokens without a nasal were included in the *uh* category (the written form <uh(m)> is used rather than <äh(m)> in order to remain consistent with the terminology used in most previous research). Tokens with slightly different vowel qualities which were clearly identical in function and comparable in form were included. Additionally, a very small number of tokens that were realised with only a nasal (/m/) were included in the *uhm* category, since in practice it was very difficult to determine a threshold for distinguishing realisations with short, reduced vowels (which can also be nasalised) followed by a nasal from those consisting of nothing but a nasal.

All annotation and coding were performed by the first author as well as a previously trained student assistant. In the very rare cases of ambiguity or disagreement regarding the coding of an utterance, both annotators discussed the issue and arrived at a unanimous solution.

For prosodic analysis of both backchannels and filled pauses, all tokens were first hand-corrected and smoothed using *Praat* (Boersma & Weenink 2021) and *mausmooth* (Cangemi 2015) (cf. the analysis of intonation styles in §3.3.2). Then, a custom *Praat* script was used to extract pitch values at 10% and 90% of token duration and the difference between those values in semitones (with a reference value of 1 Hz) was calculated, with positive values indicating pitch rises and negative values indicating falls (cf. Ha et al. 2016, Sbranna et al. 2022). Values at 10% and 90% of token duration (rather than the very first and last values) were used in order to minimise possible effects of microprosody and glottalisation that are known to occur at the extreme edges of syllables. If there was no pitch information available at either one of these time points (usually because there were unvoiced segments at the edges or because non-modal voice quality was used), the point of extraction was moved by 10%, yielding e.g. 20%–90% or 10%–80% windows. This procedure was repeated up to a maximum of 40% at the beginning and 70% at the end. The majority of pitch values, however, were extracted within 20% of start duration and 80% of end duration (>80% of tokens for BCs and 65% for FPs). Finally, all extracted values were verified through a comparison with the original extracted BC token and the smoothed pitch contour and any tokens that were unsuitable for intonational analysis were excluded. This was typically the case for tokens with a very short vocalic portion and/or those produced with creaky voice.

In the sections that follow, I will present background and results first for backchannels (§5.3) and then for filled pauses (§5.4).

5.3 Backchannels

In this section, I will present a brief overview of research on backchannels, before turning to an in-depth description of experimental results on dialogues between German dyads with and without a diagnosis of ASD.

5.3.1 Background

Backchannels (BCs) are short utterances such as *yeah* or *mmhm* whose primary function is to signal a combination of a listener's 1) understanding of, 2) attention to and 3) agreement with the interlocutor's speech. Although there is generally neither a conscious awareness of nor a formal set of rules for backchannelling, it is nevertheless a ubiquitous and essential feature of spoken communication. Backchannels have been a focus of linguistic research at least since the inception of conversation analysis in the 1970s (Clark & Schaefer 1989, Ehlich 1986, Jefferson 1984, Schegloff 1982, White 1989, Fries 1952, Birdwhistell 1962, Yngve 1970, Kendon 1967).[1]

The highly influential work of Ward & Tsukahara (2000) has highlighted the complexities of the precise prosodic, temporal and lexical realisation of backchannels and backchannel-inviting cues in English and Japanese (see also e.g. Ward 2000, 2019, Ward et al. 2007). Previous work has also shown that the rate of BCs produced and, more importantly, their specific lexical and intonational realisation, can have a profound influence on (perceived) communicative success and mutual understanding, as well as on subjective judgements by conversational partners. This has been explored both in the interactions of humans with virtual agents in spoken dialogue systems (Fujie et al. 2004, Ward & DeVault 2016, Ward & Tsukahara 1999) and in natural conversations, usually in cross-cultural or comparative settings (e.g. Cutrone 2005, 2014, Dingemanse & Liesenfeld 2022, Li 2006, Tottie 1991, Xudong 2008, Young & Lee 2004).

[1] Please note that, as mentioned elsewhere, I only focus on spoken language here, leaving aside related visual feedback signals such as eye gaze, nods and gestures, for the simple reason that conducting and analysing video recordings was note feasible at the time of data collection (see §5.7.5).

Various studies have shown that listeners are highly sensitive to the frequency and temporal placement of backchannel tokens, suggesting that unusual realisations are likely to lead to misunderstandings and negative judgements. For instance, Fujie et al. (2004) report that both the lexical content and, in particular, the timing of backchannel feedback influenced the ratings of users interacting with a robotic dialogue system. Cutrone (2005, 2014) investigated BC productions in dyadic interactions between Japanese EFL (English as a foreign language) and British speakers and concluded that between-group differences in rate, type and timing negatively affected intercultural communication. Similarly, Li (2006) found differences in the rate of BCs produced in Mandarin Chinese compared to Canadian English dialogues and, further comparing cross-cultural interactions, reports that backchannelling can be a cause for miscommunication.

Further work has analysed the prosodic realisation of backchannels in various languages in detail (Beňuš et al. 2007, Caspers 2000, Savino 2010, Stocksmeier et al. 2007). The general consensus is that BCs are typically rising in Germanic and Romance languages (but more often falling in, e.g., Japanese or Vietnamese; see Ha 2012, Ha & Grice 2010), although there are increasing hints that there is a complex interaction of this presumed "default" intonation contour with pragmatic functions and choice of lexical type (see the results in this section and subsequent related work in Sbranna et al. 2022). In a small number of pilot studies, the influence of the exact prosodic realisation of backchannels on listeners' judgements and character attributions has been explored (Ha et al. 2016, Wehrle, Roettger, et al. 2018, Wehrle & Grice 2019). Wehrle & Grice (2019) compared the intonation of BCs in German and observed that Vietnamese learners of German produced twice as many non-lexical BCs (*mmhm*) with a flat intonation contour as German natives. As discussed in Ha et al. (2016) and supported by results from a mouse-tracking experiment presented in Wehrle, Roettger, et al. (2018), a flat BC contour in German might be interpreted to signal a lack of attention or interest (see also Stocksmeier et al. 2007). These studies confirm the acute sensitivity of listeners to even small differences in the acoustic realisation of backchannel tokens.

Despite this variety of previous research, to the best of my knowledge, only two studies have touched on the topic of backchannelling in autism. The first of these studies qualitatively investigated the use of the Japanese conversational token 'ne' in highly structured interactions (in conjunction with a neuroimaging study). The authors report that 'ne' as a backchannel was not used at all by the autistic children in the sample, whereas it was used frequently by non-autistic children (Yoshimura et al. 2020). The second study analysed the use of BCs (and mutual gaze) in story-telling-based interactions and found a lower rate in autistic and mixed as compared with non-autistic dyads of adults (Rifai et al. 2022).

Although this lack of previous studies is not entirely surprising given that research on naturalistic conversations in ASD is still rare, there is a great theoretical and practical interest in further examining backchannelling in autistic populations in particular. Backchannels are implicit, other-oriented vocal signals with a predominantly social function. Given the characteristic patterns of social communication in ASD, it seems highly likely 1) that speakers with ASD might be less inclined to perform backchannelling at the same rate as non-autistic speakers (in line with previous results) and 2) that BC productions might differ in subtle ways between speakers with and without a diagnosis of ASD.

For the current study, conversations between dyads of German native speakers who either both did or did not have a diagnosis of ASD were compared. The rate of backchannels produced was analysed, taking into account different dialogue stages, as well as their lexical and prosodic realisation. The rate of BCs can indicate how much speakers explicitly supported the ongoing turn of their interlocutor, and the early stages of a social interaction are known to disproportionately influence personality judgements and character attributions (see §4.5.2.1; McAleer et al. 2014). For the analysis of the lexical realisation of backchannels, the aim was to connect the diversity of productions with the assumed general tendency towards restricted behaviour in ASD. Finally, the intonational realisation of BCs was analysed in detail, as a broad range of previous work suggests not only that prosody plays a special and potentially distinctive role in ASD (see Chapter 3 and e.g. Krüger 2018, Grice et al. 2023, McCann & Peppé 2003, Paul et al. 2005), but also that intonation may be of particular relevance in the production and perception of BCs (as pointed out above).

5.3.2 Results

In this section, I will present results first on the rate of backchannels, then on the lexical types of backchannel used and finally on their prosodic realisation. The duration of individual backchannel tokens was very consistent and practically identical across groups, with a grand mean of 375 ms (SD = 161), and will therefore not be considered in any more detail in the following.

5.3.2.1 Rate of backchannels

Overall, speakers in the ASD group produced fewer backchannels per minute of dialogue, with an average of 6.9 BCs per minute compared to the CTR group with an average of 9.2 BCs per minute. Bayesian modelling strongly suggests that this is a robust difference between groups (see below).

Analysis at the dyad-level confirms the impression from the group-level analysis. The four lowest mean values of backchannels per minute were produced by autistic dyads (the lowest rate being 3 BCs per minute), while three out of the four highest mean values were produced by non-autistic dyads (including the highest rate, 12.3 BCs per minute); see Figure 5.1. Please note that, once more, these data do not suggest a clear dividing line between the behaviour of autistic and non-autistic dyads. They instead reveal a considerable degree of overlap between groups. For instance, although the ASD group as a whole clearly produced fewer backchannels per minute, the dyad with the second-highest overall rate was part of the ASD group.

Data were considered only at the level of the dyad, not the level of the individual, for this analysis, as the rate of backchannelling fundamentally depends on the behaviour of the interlocutor and their production of silences and backchannel-inviting cues, among other factors (and because interlocutors should not be treated as independent by default due to factors such as accommodation to the conversational partner; see e.g. results in §5.4.2.1 and Winter & Grice 2021).

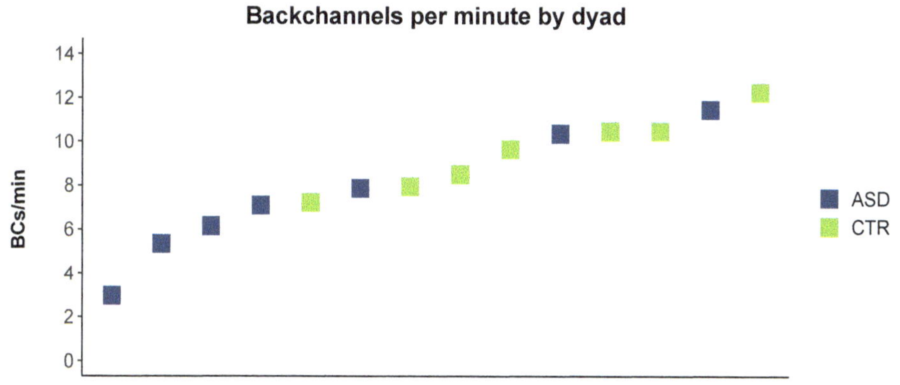

Figure 5.1: Rate of backchannels produced per minute of dialogue by dyad. ASD group in blue, CTR group in green.

The group difference in the rate of BCs per minute of dialogue was not dependent on different overall amounts of speech produced: as has already been established (§4.4.4.2), extremely similar proportions of silence, single-speaker speech and overlapping speech were produced by both groups. A related way of corroborating this finding is to calculate the rate of BCs not per minute of dialogue but per minute of speech produced within a dialogue (i.e. excluding all stretches of silence). This analysis yields an almost identical finding to the above, with a lower rate for the ASD (9.1) compared with the CTR group (11.8). In other words, the CTR group produced about 1.3 times more backchannels than the ASD group, regardless of whether the rate of BCs per minute of dialogue or per minute of speech is considered.

Bayesian modelling

A Bayesian model was fitted to the rate of backchannels per minute using negative binomial regression. Negative binomial regression is a more robust extension of Poisson regression. The Poisson distribution is the canonical distribution for characterising count data (Winter & Bürkner 2021). Both negative binomial regression and Poisson regression were tested and the negative binomial model was found to perform better. Negative binomial regression is also usually the more conservative choice and thereby reduces the chance of Type I errors (Winter & Bürkner 2021).

The input for the model was a data frame with one row per dyad containing columns to specify the overall count of backchannels and the duration of the respective dialogue. Total number of backchannels was used as the dependent variable, with group as the independent variable and dialogue duration as the offset (or exposure variable).

Bayesian modelling supports the observation that there was a difference between groups of autistic and non-autistic dyads. Model estimates show a lower rate of BCs per minute for ASD dyads ($\hat{\beta} = 7.39$, CI = [5.72, 9.57]) than for CTR dyads ($\hat{\beta} = 9.64$, CI = [7.47, 12.45]).

The group difference in the model is reported with the ASD group as the reference level. Mean $\delta = 2.25$, indicating a higher rate of BCs in the CTR group. The 95% CI [-0.22, 4.88] includes zero by a small margin and the posterior probability $P(\delta > 0)$ is 0.94. Although these values reflect a more than negligible degree of uncertainty, the overall tendency towards a higher rate of backchannels in non-autistic speakers is very strong. At the very least, we can conclude that, based on the model, the data and prior beliefs, it is far more probable that the difference between groups is a robust effect.

Regularising weakly informative priors with a normal distribution were specified for the intercept ($\mu = 0, \delta = 12$) and for the regression coefficient ($\mu = 0, \delta = 3$) and used the default priors of the *brms* package for the shape parameter ($\gamma = 0.01$).

Stage of dialogue

For the comparison of dialogue stages, resolution of the first Mismatch was used as the cut-off point. Detection of the first Mismatch was not used simply because for many dyads there was not enough backchannel data available prior to detection of the first Mismatch to allow for a reliable comparison (five dyads produced only seven BCs or less prior to detection of the first Mismatch; see also §2.2, §4.4.1.3 and §4.4.1.4 for definition and analysis of dialogue stages).

At the group level, the pattern of the ASD group producing fewer backchannels is shown to be very robust for the early stages of dialogue, but not for the remainder; see Figure 5.2. Specifically, in the first few minutes of dialogue, the ASD group produced an average rate of 5.8 backchannels per minute and the CTR group produced an average rate of 9.8 backchannels per minute (δ = 4). In the remainder of the dialogue, rates were more similar between groups, with the ASD group producing an average rate of 7.2 backchannels per minute and the CTR group producing an average rate of 8.6 (δ = 1.4).

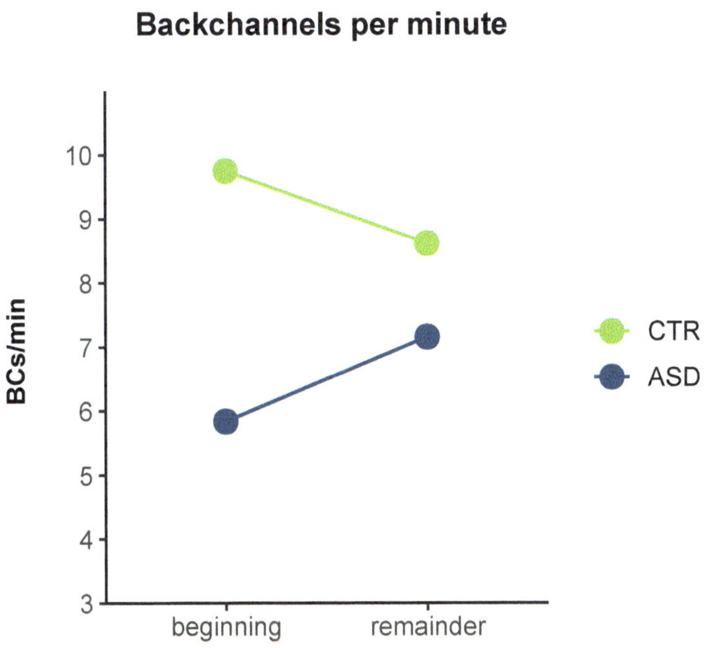

Figure 5.2: Rate of backchannels per minute by dialogue stage (before and after resolution of the first Mismatch). CTR group in green, ASD group in blue.

Bayesian modelling clearly confirms the difference between groups in the early stages of dialogue, but not in the remainder. Differences between groups are presented with the ASD group as the reference level. Before resolution of the first Mismatch, mean δ = 3.9, with a 95% CI of [0.9, 7.13] and a posterior probability $P(\delta > 0)$ of 0.98. This reflects a robust difference, with a higher rate of BCs in the CTR group

After resolution of the first Mismatch, mean δ = 1.89, with a 95% CI of [-1.01, 4.89] and a posterior probability $P(\delta > 0)$ of 0.87. This is indicative of the same trend as for the early dialogue stage, but does not signify a robust difference between groups. This model contained dyad as a random factor, which was not included in the model for the dialogue as a whole, as in that case there was only one observation per dyad.

At the dyad level, we can see that a high degree of variability underlies the group-level results, particularly in the ASD group, where by-dyad variability was much greater than in the CTR group; see Figure 5.3. To compare rates in the beginning and the remainder of the dialogue, ratios were calculated, such that a ratio of two, for instance, represents twice as many backchannels *after* resolution of the first Mismatch.

For all CTR dyads (bottom row in Figure 5.3), the rate of backchannels was similar throughout the conversation, represented in ratios ranging from 0.78 to 1.19. In this group, two dyads produced almost exactly the same rate throughout (with ratios of 1 and 1.05, respectively), one dyad produced fewer backchannels in the beginning and three dyads produced more backchannels in the beginning (see Table C.1 in Appendix C for ratios by dyad).

ASD dyads (top row in Figure 5.3) lie at the edges of the overall distribution, with all of them producing either higher or lower ratios than any non-autistic dyad. Ratios ranged from 0.64 to 2.78. No dyad produced the same (or nearly the same) rate of backchannels throughout, four dyads produced fewer backchannels in the beginning and three dyads produced more backchannels in the beginning. It is important to note that the group level pattern is thus representative only of the behaviour of a little more than half of all autistic dyads.

Speaker roles

In the analysis of speaker roles, rather than calculating rates of backchannel per minute of dialogue, the relative duration of backchannels in proportion to the duration of all speech produced (excluding silence) was calculated. A comparison based on overall dialogue duration would not be informative as it fails to

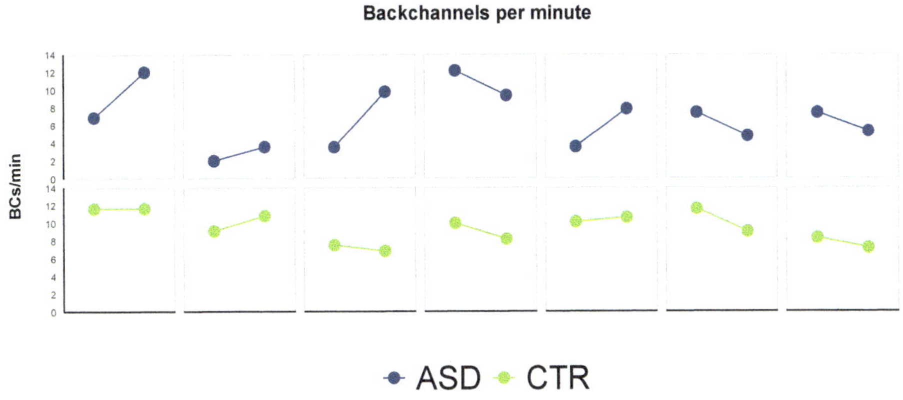

Figure 5.3: Rate of backchannels per minute by dialogue stage (before and after resolution of the first Mismatch) and dyad. The left dot in each panel represents the rate for the beginning of the dialogue, the right dot the rate for the remainder. ASD dyads on top and in blue, CTR dyads on the bottom and in green.

acknowledge the fact that instruction followers produced far less speech overall than instruction givers.

As backchannels are specifically a signal produced by the listener, it is not surprising that instruction followers produced a much higher proportion of backchannels than givers, in both the ASD group (followers: 11.2%; givers: 2.1%) and in the CTR group (followers: 14.5%; givers: 3.4%). A by-dyad analysis confirms this pattern while once again highlighting the greater variability in the ASD group.

5.3.2.2 Lexical realisation

In this section, the frequency of occurrence for different lexical types of BC is examined. Backchannel tokens were divided into four main categories: *genau* ('exactly'), *ja* ('yes/yeah'), *okay* and finally what I refer to as *non-lexical* backchannels and transcribed *mmhm*. The vast majority of the tokens in the *mmhm* category were produced with two energy peaks, leading to their perception as 'disyllabic' and corresponding to the orthographic form of the chosen category label, ⟨mmhm⟩. Although the remaining tokens only had one clear energy peak each, being closer in realisation to what might be transcribed as ⟨mm⟩ (or described as monosyllabic), they were subsumed under the same category of *mmhm* as there is no clear and categorical distinction between these two types of phonetic realisation, but rather a continuum, and because the /mmhm/ realisation (with two peaks) was far more frequent overall.

The four main categories (*genau, ja, mmhm, okay*) cover 91.8% of all backchannel tokens in the data set. All remaining tokens were classified as *other*. The most frequent types of BC in this *other* category were *gut* ('good/fine'), *alles klar* ('alright') and *richtig/korrekt/exakt* ('right/correct/exactly'), in descending order of frequency.

Results at the group level show that choice of backchannel type was very similar between groups overall; see Figure 5.4. The most commonly used BC type in both groups was *ja* ('yes/yeah'), with proportions of 47.7% (ASD; n = 336) and 44% (CTR; n = 733), respectively. The second most frequent BC type differed between groups. The ASD group showed a stronger preference for *mmhm* (25.6%; n = 180) than the CTR group (16.5%; n = 275), but in turn produced fewer *okay* tokens (11.6%; n = 82) than the CTR group (20.5%; n = 341). The remainder was made up of tokens from the *genau* (ASD: 7.4% (n = 52); CTR: 10.7% (n = 178)) and *other* categories (ASD: 7.7% (n = 54); CTR: 8.4% (n = 140)).

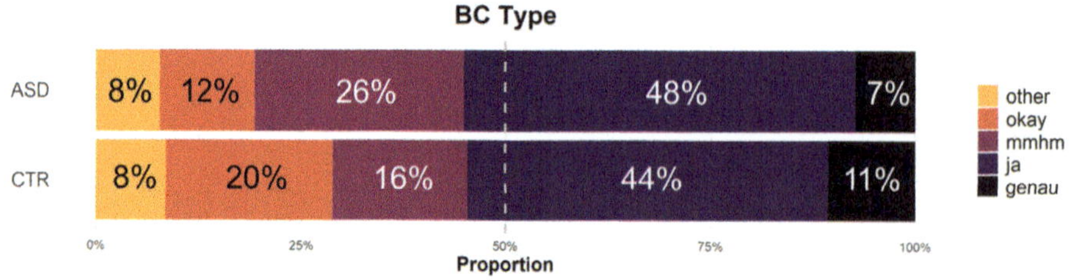

Figure 5.4: Stacked bar charts by group showing proportions of different backchannel types. ASD group on top, CTR group below.

Analysis at the level of the individual reveals some intriguing speaker-specific variation that also has implications for the group comparison, but is hidden when only considering proportions averaged across speakers within a group. The general trends seen in the group analysis are clearly reflected in the behaviour of individual speakers and the choice of backchannel type remained similar across groups. We can observe, however, that half of the ASD speakers used a narrower *range* of BC types and showed clearer preferences for particular BC types over others, compared to CTR speakers. These differences will be described first in absolute terms and then using Shannon entropy as a measure of diversity.

All 14 speakers from the CTR group used all five categories of BCs (see overview plot in Figure C.1 in Appendix C). This was not the case for the ASD group, in which only 7 out of 14 speakers used BCs from all five categories, and only 9 speakers used BCs from all four main categories (excluding *other*). Additionally,

ASD speakers accounted for six out of the seven clearest individual preferences. For instance, speaker M10A produced 75% *ja* (n = 75) and two speakers from the same dyad (M04_M05) both produced 69% *ja* (M04: n = 40; M05: n = 24). In contrast, most CTR speakers used a fairly even mixture of different BCs. Overall, 11 out of 28 speakers used just one type of BC for 50% or more of all BC tokens produced, and 8 out of these 11 speakers (72%) were part of the ASD group.

Entropy as a measure of backchannel diversity

While the above pattern of results can be understood quite well through description and visualisation alone, this approach does not provide us with any quantifiable measure of how diverse the production of different backchannel types actually was for individual speakers or by group. (The focus here is on speakers rather than dyads for the sake of clarity, but it was verified that analysis at the dyad level yields equivalent results.) The measure of Shannon entropy can be used as an index of diversity for this purpose (Shannon 1948). The higher the value of entropy (H), the more diverse the signal.

To give two extreme examples from the data set under investigation, Speaker M13 from the CTR group had the highest entropy value ($H = 2.23$); see Figure 5.5. Like all non-autistic speakers, M13 produced backchannels from all five categories, and in this specific case, there was no strong preference for any one type. The least frequent category was *mmhm*, with 13.3% (n = 16), and the most frequent category was *ja*, with 34.3% (n = 36). This high degree of diversity or, in other words, less predictable behaviour, is reflected in a higher entropy value.

By contrast, speaker M10A from the ASD group had the lowest entropy value of all speakers ($H = 1.18$). Interestingly, this speaker in fact belonged to the 50% of individuals from the ASD group who *did* use BCs from all five categories. However, tokens were far from evenly spread out among these categories. M10A used *ja* in 75% of cases (n = 75), followed by *mmhm* with a proportion of 14% (n = 14), as shown in Figure 5.5. Such a clear preference for one type of backchannel corresponds to a lower degree of diversity, or in other words, more predictable behaviour, and is reflected in a lower entropy value.

Entropy values for all 28 speakers are shown in Figure 5.6, revealing a clear pattern of higher entropy values for non-autistic speakers overall. Note that while in this case there is a fairly clear separation between groups, there is still overlap between them. For instance, several autistic speakers have very high values of entropy and one non-autistic speaker has the second lowest entropy value overall.

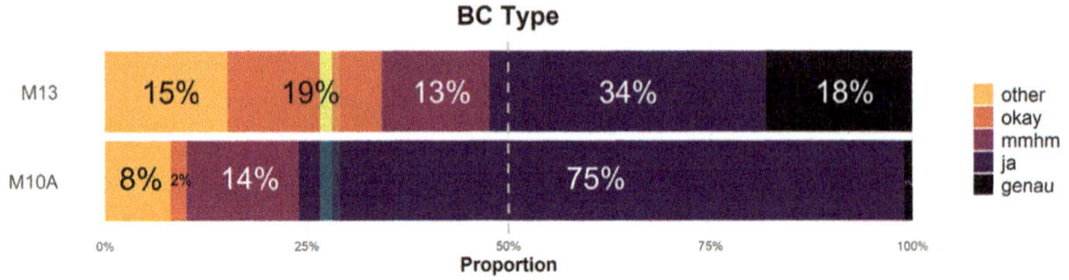

Figure 5.5: Stacked bar charts showing proportions of different backchannel types for the two speakers with the highest entropy value (M13, CTR group; $H = 2.23$) and the lowest entropy value (M10A, ASD group; $H = 1.18$), respectively.

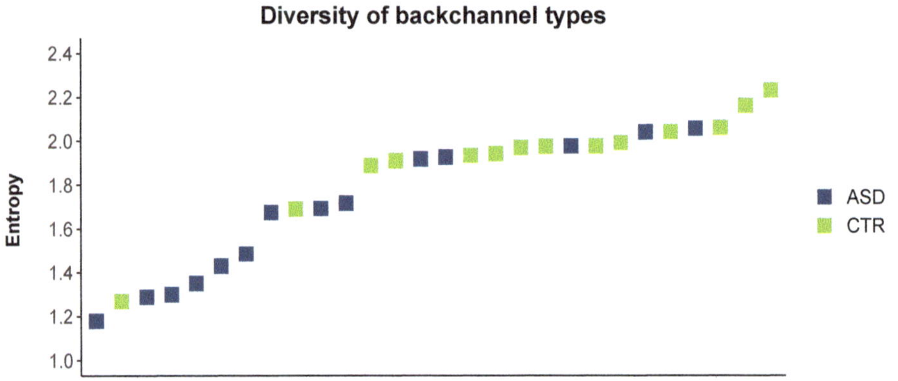

Figure 5.6: Entropy as a measure of the diversity of lexical types of backchannel produced, by speaker. ASD group in blue, CTR group in green.

Bayesian modelling confirms that backchannels were more diverse in the CTR group. A Bayesian model was fitted to entropy values by speaker using a log-normal distribution. Model output shows that the difference between groups is robust, in showing a lower estimated entropy value for the ASD group ($\hat{\beta} = 1.68$, CI = [1.53, 1.81]) than for the CTR group ($\hat{\beta} = 1.88$, CI = [1.73, 2.04]).

The group difference in the model is reported with the ASD group as the reference level. Mean $\delta = 0.21$, indicating higher entropy in the CTR group. The 95% CI [0.05, 0.38] does not include zero and the posterior probability $P(\delta > 0)$ is 0.99. The lower end of the 95% credible interval is relatively close to 0, but because values are generally low (the maximum possible entropy value would be 2.32) and and the posterior probability is very high, this can be considered as compelling evidence for the observation that CTR speakers were more diverse in their production of BC types than ASD speakers.

Regularising weakly informative priors with a normal distribution were specified for the intercept ($\mu = 0$, $\delta = 0.5$) and for the regression coefficient ($\mu = 0$, $\delta = 0.3$) and used the default priors of the *brms* package for the standard deviation of the likelihood function, Student's *t*-distribution ($\nu = 3$, $\mu = 0$, $\delta = 2.5$).

Speaker roles and dialogue stages

The choice of backchannel type was consistent throughout conversations for both groups. In other words, proportions of backchannel types were the same for all stages of dialogue within each group.

Considering speaker roles, however, revealed some interesting differences in the way backchannels were used by instruction followers compared to instruction givers; see Figure 5.7. For example, *genau* ('exactly') was used far more frequently in the speech of instruction givers compared with followers (ASD: followers 2.3% – givers 21.5%; CTR: followers 5% – givers 23.5%; see black bars in Figure 5.7). This was compensated for with a decrease of *ja* ('yes/yeah') and *mmhm*, while the proportion of *okay* remained more or less constant. This pattern holds true for the majority of individual speakers in both groups.

The most obvious explanation for this finding is that the backchannel token *genau* ('exactly') is likely to be a semantically appropriate choice in many cases for a speaker who possesses, provides and, crucially, confirms information regarding the route and landmarks, but less so for an instruction follower (and vice versa for the non-lexical BC type *mmhm*).

5.3.2.3 Intonational realisation

As described in §5.2 above, all backchannel tokens were hand-corrected and smoothed before undergoing prosodic analysis. No sufficient pitch information for prosodic analysis could be extracted for 302 tokens; these were usually rather short and/or produced with non-modal voice quality. After careful inspection of the extracted pitch contours for the remaining tokens, a further 20 tokens that were not suitable for intonational analysis were excluded (most of these were produced with very creaky voice). Following this step, 2069 BC tokens remained for analysis (87.3% of the original 2371). It is interesting to note that there was a far lower proportion of the usually disyllabic and fully voiced *mmhm* type (5%) in the subset of excluded tokens than in the full data set, reflecting the fact that the other lexical types (e.g. *okay*) are inherently more susceptible to being realised

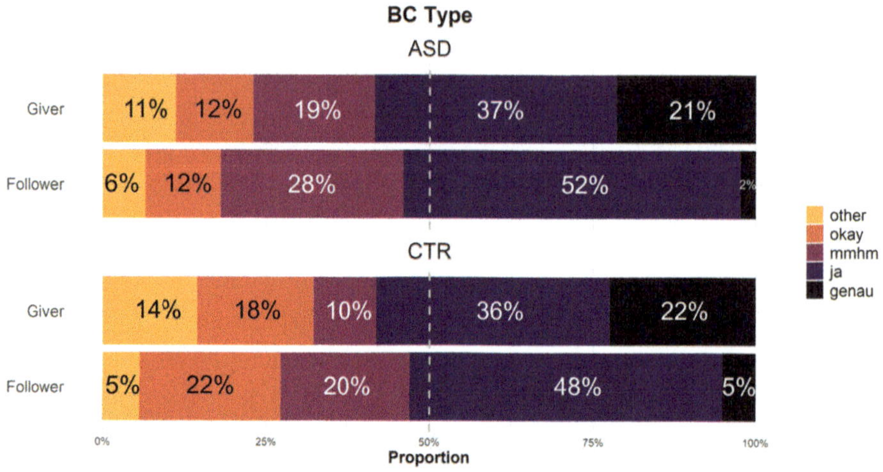

Figure 5.7: Stacked bar charts by group and role showing proportions of different backchannel types. For each group, instruction givers are displayed above instruction followers. ASD group in the top panel, CTR group in the bottom panel.

in forms with reduced periodic energy, which in turn makes such realisations problematic for prosodic analysis.

Finally, all tokens that were not part of the four main categories (*ja, mmhm, okay, genau*) were excluded. This necessitated the exclusion of a further 137 tokens, leaving a total of 1932 tokens (81.4% of the original 2371). This step was taken because prosodic realisation was analysed separately for different lexical types of BC. As we shall see, speakers used very specific mappings for different backchannel types, thereby greatly reducing the utility of a monolithic analysis across different types.

I will first describe a continuous analysis, then a categorical view in which realisations were split up into the three categories of rising, falling and level pitch contours (more information in §5.3.2.3). The categorical analysis not only facilitates detecting and describing overarching patterns of prosodic realisation, but also makes it possible to explicitly account for the potentially distinct status of level (or flat) intonation contours (see §5.4; cf. Grice et al. 2017, Sbranna et al. 2022).

Speaker roles and different stages within dialogues did not have any major effects on intonational realisation. There was a slight tendency for more falling contours in the later stages of dialogue across groups and BC types. Similarly, there was a slight overall tendency for more falling contours in the speech of instruction givers compared with followers across groups and BC types. However, as these effects were weak and not consistent across speakers, they will be disregarded in the following analyses.

Continuous analysis

Figure 5.8 shows violin (and scatter) plots of intonation contours by backchannel type and across groups. Values are shown across groups in order to emphasise the differences between lexical types of backchannel. Group differences will be analysed separately for each type in the following section. Across groups, intonation greatly differed according to backchannel type. For instance, *mmhm* tokens were produced almost entirely with rising intonation by both groups of speakers, while there was a clear preference for falling intonation contours on *genau* for both groups.

An analysis by group and lexical type reveals that there were between-group differences in intonational realisation for all lexical types except *mmhm*. Figure 5.9 and Table 5.1 show mean ST values for pitch movement and standard deviations by group and backchannel type.

Table 5.1: Intonational realisation of BCs by type and group. Negative values indicate falling contours; positive values indicate rising contours. ST = semitones; SD = standard deviation.

		Contour (ST)	
BC Type	Group	Mean	SD
genau	ASD	-4.30	5.65
genau	CTR	-2.53	5.13
ja	ASD	3.15	4.26
ja	CTR	1.74	3.67
mmhm	ASD	5.70	4.27
mmhm	CTR	5.98	3.64
okay	ASD	1.38	5.70
okay	CTR	-0.63	4.89

Bayesian linear regression modelling confirms that there were robust group differences in the intonational realisation of three out of the four BC types (*okay*, *ja* and *genau*). In contrast, there was clearly no difference between groups for *mmhm*, recalling the special status of this non-lexical BC type and reflecting

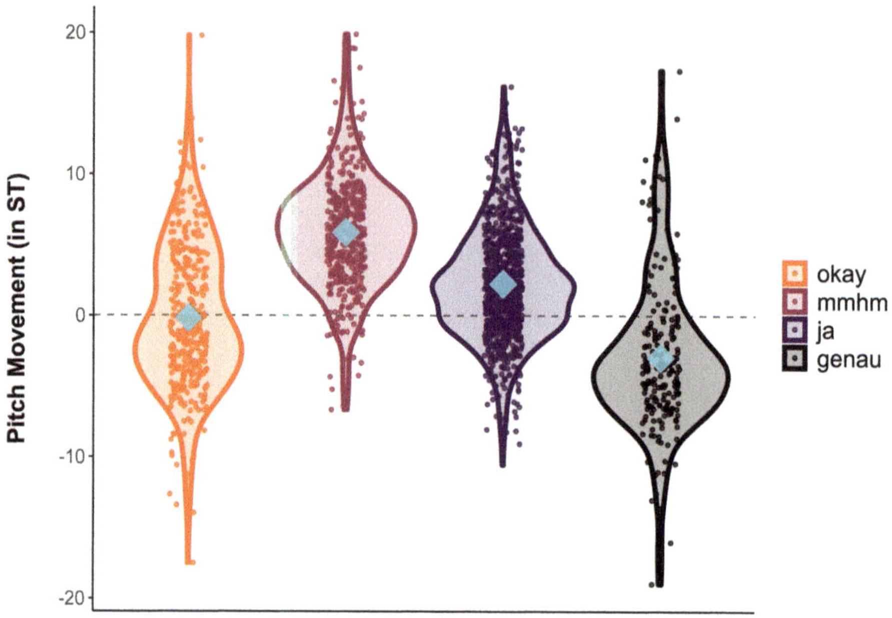

Figure 5.8: Intonational realisation of backchannels by type in semitones (pooled across speakers and groups). Negative values indicate falling contours; positive values indicate rising contours. Blue diamonds represent mean values.

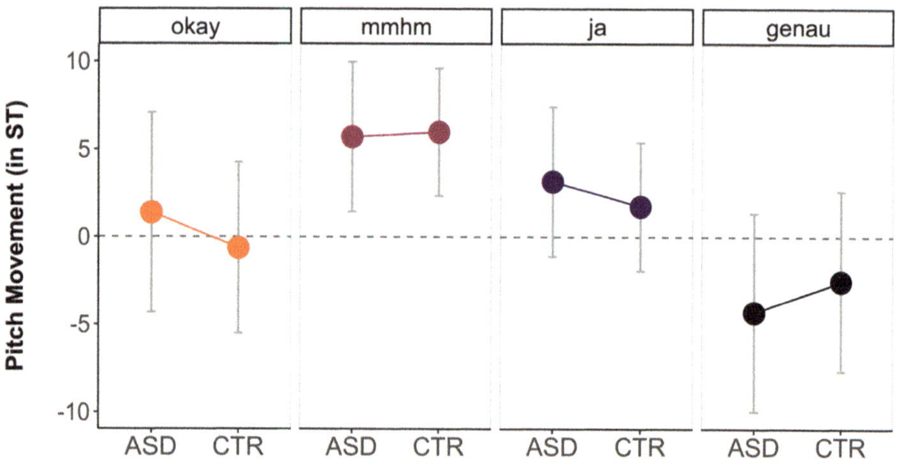

Figure 5.9: Mean values (dots) and SD (error bars) for intonation contours, by backchannel type and group. ASD group on the left side of each panel, CTR group on the right side of each panel.

the fact that almost all *mmhm* tokens were realised with rises, in both groups. Model results are summarised below by BC type. More details can be found in the accompanying scripts and files (see https://osf.io/jcb7t/).

For *okay*, mean δ = -2.2 (ST), indicating more falling and fewer rising contours in the CTR group. The 95% CI [-4.16, -0.19] does not include zero and the posterior probability $P(\delta > 0)$ is 0.96. This indicates that there war a robust difference between groups in the intonational realisation of *okay* BCs.

For *mmhm*, mean δ = 0.49, the 95% CI is [-1.33, 2.29] and the posterior probability $P(\delta > 0)$ is 0.67. This clearly shows that there was no robust group difference in the intonational realisation of *mmhm* tokens.

For *ja*, mean δ = -2.03, indicating more falling and fewer rising contours in the CTR group. The 95% CI [-3.37, -0.67] does not include zero and the posterior probability $P(\delta > 0)$ is 0.99. This very clearly indicates that there was a robust difference between groups in the intonational realisation of *ja* BCs.

For *genau*, mean δ = 1.77, indicating more rising and fewer falling contours in the CTR group. The 95% CI is [-0.06, 3.54] and the posterior probability $P(\delta > 0)$ is 0.95. Although the CI includes zero by a very narrow margin, this model output still very strongly favours the interpretation that there was a robust group difference in the intonational realisation of *genau* tokens.

Categorical analysis

For the categorical analysis of intonation, all contours with pitch movement within the range of ±1 semitone were counted as *level* (i.e. all tokens with absolute values ≤1). An absolute pitch difference of 1 semitone is somewhat greater than the thresholds of "just noticeable" pitch differences reported in some recent experimental studies (Jongman et al. 2017, Liu 2013), but considerably smaller than the values proposed in 't Hart (1981). In any case, auditory inspection of all tokens in the relevant range confirmed that pitch movement was subtle at most and that the extracted values accurately reflected the original intonation contours.

Figure 5.10 shows the proportions of falling, level and rising pitch contours by group and backchannel type, and confirms that 1) differences between groups were subtle and 2) intonational realisation varied greatly by BC type. In other words, there was a specific, albeit probabilistic mapping of intonation contours to different types of backchannel for both the ASD and the CTR group. The only difference between groups noticeable at this level of analysis is a stronger overall preference for rising backchannels in the ASD group. Averaging across backchannel types, 67.6% (n = 427) of contours were rises in the ASD group, compared to

54% (n = 702) in the CTR group. This pattern will be elucidated in the following through detailed analyses of speaker-specific behaviour and of the diversity of intonation contours produced.

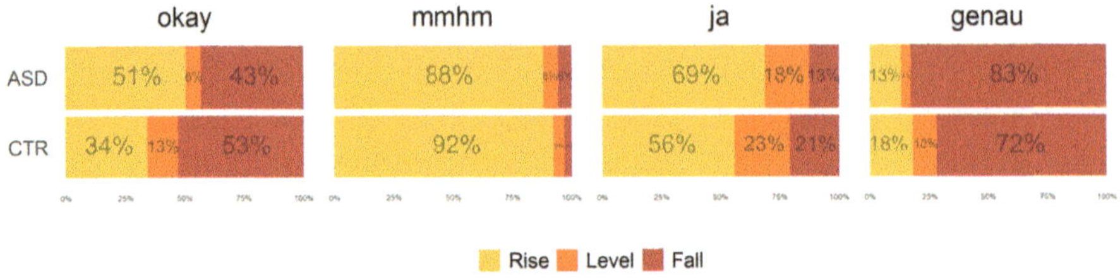

Figure 5.10: Intonation contour by group and backchannel type. Rising contours in yellow, level contours in orange and falling contours in red. Level contours were defined as all tokens with a pitch difference in the range of ±1 semitone.

Speaker-specific analysis of the intonational realisation of backchannels reveals firstly that the behaviour of the CTR group was more homogeneous overall than that of the ASD group (as was the case for many other measures reported in this book). The individual distributions of almost all non-autistic speakers matched the averaged group distribution to an almost uncanny degree, as shown in Figure 5.11 (bottom two rows). This was not the case for the ASD group (uppermost rows). Besides the fact that 5 out of 14 autistic speakers did not produce backchannels from all four main categories (whereas all non-autistic speakers used all categories), many speakers also do not show evidence for the precise mapping of intonation contour to backchannel type that is evident at the group level. Instead, around half of all autistic speakers used predominantly rising contours *regardless* of backchannel type.

The relevance and robustness of the diversity of such distributions can be quantitatively analysed using the measure of Shannon entropy (as for the analysis of lexical types in §5.3.2.2). An entropy value (H) of 0 signifies that all backchannels of a category were produced with the same intonation contour, while the maximum entropy value in this case is 1.58 (equal proportions for all three types of contour). At the group level, entropy was higher for the CTR group across backchannels and also for each individual BC type except *mmhm*. For a more representative, in-depth analysis, entropy was also calculated by speaker (and BC type). Results confirm that entropy was higher on average for non-autistic speakers in all categories except *mmhm*. Results by group are shown in Table 5.2 and results by speaker are shown in Figure 5.12.

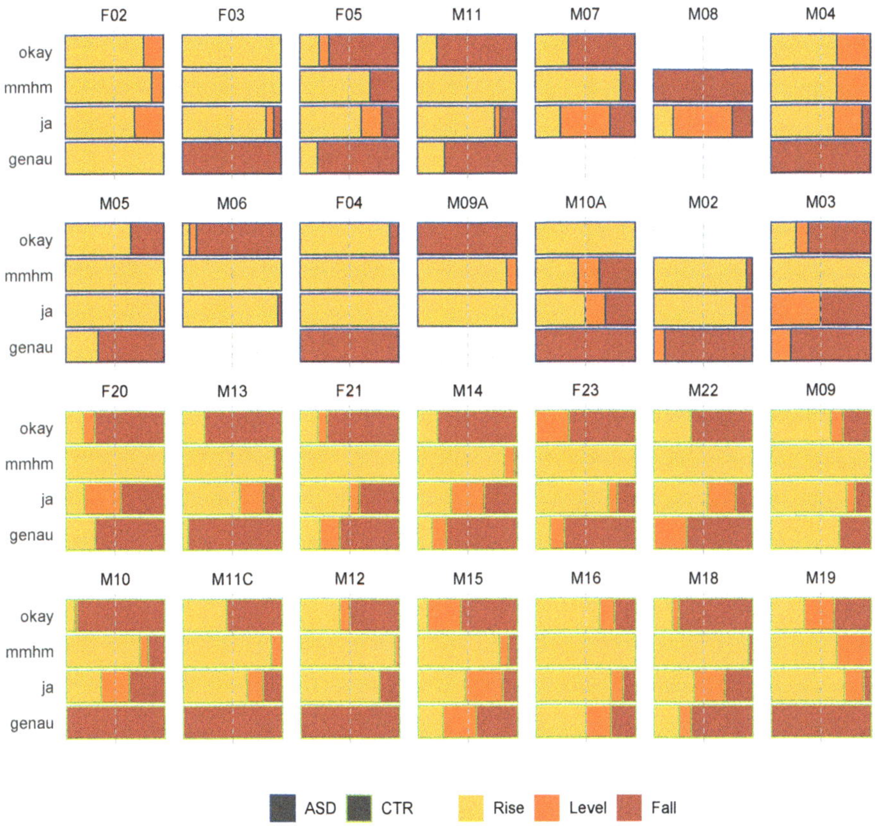

Figure 5.11: Intonation contour by speaker and backchannel type. ASD speakers in the top two rows and with blue outlines, CTR speakers in the bottom two rows and with green outlines. Rising contours in yellow, level contours in orange and falling contours in red. Level contours were defined as all tokens with a pitch difference in the range of ±1 semitone.

The non-lexical backchannel *mmhm* stands out by having a lower entropy value. This is because, as observed above, it was realised with a rising contour in the vast majority of cases. This held true for all but two speakers (M08 and M10A, both from the ASD group).

Table 5.2: Shannon entropy (*H*), measuring the diversity of intonation contours, by BC type and group.

BC Type	Group	H
genau	ASD	0.80
genau	CTR	1.13
ja	ASD	1.20
ja	CTR	1.43
mmhm	ASD	0.64
mmhm	CTR	0.46
okay	ASD	1.27
okay	CTR	1.40

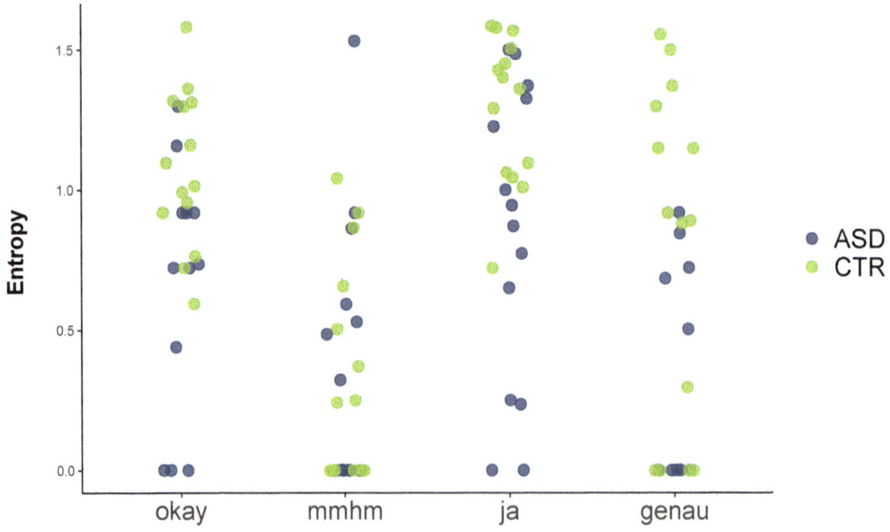

Figure 5.12: Entropy as a measure of the diversity of intonation contours, by speaker and backchannel type. ASD group in blue, CTR group in green.

Bayesian modelling confirms these group differences as robust except in the case of the non-lexical backchannel type *mmhm*. Details are reported in the following paragraphs.

Entropy values by speaker were fitted to four separate Bayesian models, one for each main type of backchannel. All models used a skew normal distribution. While log-normal distributions were used for Bayesian models of entropy elsewhere, this was not suitable in this case as the data contained a number of data points with entropy values of 0 (where all backchannels were produced with the same type of contour). A hurdle log-normal distribution can be used in such cases, but skew-normal distributions provided a considerably better fit in every instance. The ASD group was used as the reference level for the group comparison. Results for the difference between groups for each backchannel type in turn are reported below. For further details, see scripts and files in the accompanying repository.

For *okay*, mean $\delta = 0.36$, indicating higher entropy values in the CTR group. The 95% CI [0.12, 0.63] does not include zero and the posterior probability $P(\delta > 0)$ is 0.99. This confirms that intonation contours were less diverse for autistic speakers (many of whom used predominantly rises for *okay*).

For *mmhm*, mean $\delta = 0$, indicating no difference whatsoever between groups. The 95% CI [-0.17, 0.17] is centered at zero and the posterior probability $P(\delta > 0)$ is 0.51. This unequivocally shows that there was no difference between groups (most speakers across groups produced at least 80% rises on *mmhm*).

For *ja*, mean $\delta = 0.26$, indicating higher entropy values in the CTR group. The 95% CI [0.03, 0.57] does not include zero and the posterior probability $P(\delta > 0)$ is 0.97. This confirms that intonation contours were less diverse for autistic speakers (most of whom showed a clear preference for rises). Please note that the lower end of the credible interval is very close to zero, meaning that results should be interpreted with at least a certain amount of caution here.

For *genau*, mean $\delta = 0.41$, indicating higher entropy values in the CTR group. The 95% CI is [0, 0.77] and the posterior probability $P(\delta > 0)$ is 0.95. This confirms that intonation contours were less diverse for autistic speakers (most of whom showed a clear preference for falls – or produced no *genau* tokens at all). Please note that as the lower end of the credible interval just includes zero, results should be interpreted with a certain degree of caution.

5.3.3 Summary

This in-depth analysis of backchannel productions has yielded a number of insights, both at a general level and specifically for the comparison of dialogues by autistic and non-autistic dyads. First, it was found that ASD dyads produced fewer backchannels per minute than CTR dyads and that this effect was particularly clear in the early stages of dialogue (cf. the similar pattern for turn-timing described in §4.4.1.3). It was also shown that instruction followers produced a far higher rate of backchannels than instruction givers (across groups).

Second, an analysis of lexical realisation revealed that *ja* ('yes/yeah') was by the far most common type across groups, but that groups differed in the diversity of their BC productions. In other words, ASD speakers showed clearer preferences for certain BC types and used a smaller range of different BC types, whereas all CTR speakers employed BCs from all five lexical categories and spread tokens out more evenly across these different categories. It was also shown that speaker roles influenced the choice of BC type, with e.g. instruction givers using considerably more *genau* ('exactly') than instruction followers.

Third, prosodic analysis revealed a number of interesting patterns. Across groups, intonation contours were (probabilistically) mapped onto specific backchannel types, with e.g. *mmhm* produced almost exclusively with rising intonation and *genau* ('exactly') produced predominantly with falling intonation. Both the continuous and the categorical analysis of backchannel intonation showed that ASD speakers and CTR speakers differed in their prosodic realisations, with many ASD speakers e.g. preferring rises regardless of BC type, reflecting a less flexible mapping of intonation contours to BC types.

It bears repeating that these patterns held true for most but not all speakers, and that there was considerable overlap between groups.

5.4 Filled pauses

This section will first provide a synopsis of research on filled pauses in conversation and then a description of the results on data from dialogue between German dyads with and without a diagnosis of autism spectrum disorder. The subsequent sections report on analyses of the role of silent pauses, of the interaction between filled pauses and following stretches of silence, and of laughter.

5.4.1 Background

Similarly to backchannels, filled pauses such as *uh(m)* are a ubiquitous feature of spoken interaction. Functionally, however, they are the polar opposite, as they are typically used to signal hesitation or uncertainty (rather than understanding and agreement) and are intended to help the current speaker hold the floor, or sometimes to take over the floor from the interlocutor (rather than supporting their ongoing turn) (Belz 2021, Beňuš 2009, Fischer 2000, Schettino 2019, Shriberg 2001, Ward 2006). Another similarity to backchannels is that filled pauses, too, are rarely, if ever, produced consciously and deliberately. In contrast to backchannels, the use of which is usually either ignored or encouraged, producing filled pauses has often been judged and perceived to be undesirable, with certain educational and training settings actually aiming to eradicate their use, at least in formal, monologic speech (Erard 2008, Fischer 2013, Fox Tree 2002, Niebuhr & Fischer 2019, O'Connell & Kowal 2004, Smith & Clark 1993, Ward 2019).

Although a higher rate of filled pauses can lead to more negative judgements in the specific case of public speaking (Niebuhr & Fischer 2019), filled pauses in dialogue actually facilitate understanding and aid the flow of conversation. Filled pauses can serve a range of crucial functions in conversation, e.g. signalling politeness and attention or foreshadowing the duration and informativeness of upcoming linguistic elements, which aids in the planning and processing of complex utterances (Corley & Hartsuiker 2003, Fox Tree 2001, Fruehwald 2016, Levinson 1983, Niebuhr & Fischer 2019, Schegloff 2010).

I will focus on the two most common types of filled pause (by far), those realised either with only a central vowel (*uh*) or a central vowel followed by a nasal (*uhm*). Although similar in segmental form, a number of studies have found important differences between *uh* and *uhm*, suggesting e.g. that *uh* is perceived more negatively than *uhm* (Niebuhr & Fischer 2019) and that *uhm* is not only more frequent than *uh*, but is also continuing to gain ground in an ongoing process of linguistic change (Fruehwald 2016, Wieling et al. 2016). Some authors have further proposed that *uhm* might be functionally different from *uh*. *Uhm* not only seems to reliably cue longer silent pauses than *uh* (Clark & Fox Tree 2002, Fox Tree 2001) – a finding which I have examined and attempted to replicate separately; see §5.5 – but it has also been suggested that *uhm* might be a more specifically listener-oriented conversational signal than *uh* (Gorman et al. 2016, Irvine et al. 2016, McGregor & Hadden 2020).

It is important to note at this point that all of these specific aspects of filled pause production can only safely be assumed to apply to West Germanic languages, as most studies used data from German, English or Dutch (for which results are very similar). A number of studies from other language families show that, while a distinction between two filled pause types – one consisting of only a vowel and the other with the addition of a final nasal – is very common, there are differences in their exact phonetic realisation, especially in terms of vowel quality (Anansiripinyo & Onsuwan 2019, Di Napoli 2020, Kosmala & Crible 2022,

Nguyễn 2015, Schettino 2019, Yuan et al. 2016). There also seems to be a differential (possibly increased) use of other forms of hesitation such as repetition and prolongation in other languages, and particularly in tone languages (Betz et al. 2017, Lee et al. 2004, Tseng 2003).

Regarding prosodic realisation, there is abundant, cross-linguistic evidence that filled pauses are typically produced with flat or level intonation contours, and that they tend to be relatively low in pitch (Adell et al. 2010, Belz & Reichel 2015, O'Shaughnessy 1992, Shriberg & Lickley 1993). The current study is the first to consider prosodic aspects of filled pauses in ASD.

5.4.1.1 Previous work on filled pauses in autism

Research on the use of filled pauses by speakers on the autism spectrum is limited, but growing. To my awareness, there are eight previous studies focussing on filled pauses in ASD, none of which analysed conversations between autistic adults (as in the current work). Seven out of these eight studies analysed the speech of children or adolescents (Gorman et al. 2016, Irvine et al. 2016, Jones et al. 2022, Lunsford et al. 2010, McGregor & Hadden 2020, Parish-Morris et al. 2017, Suh et al. 2014), while one analysed the speech of autistic adults interacting with a – presumably non-autistic – experimenter (Lake et al. 2011). Most studies analysed speech that was either monologic or produced in the context of structured interviews with a trained professional (with the exception of Jones et al. 2022: here, semi-structured double interviews were used), in many cases through use of the autism diagnostic observation schedule (ADOS) (Lord et al. 2000).

All studies but one (Suh et al. 2014) found differences between the filled pause productions of autistic and non-autistic participants (but see also related results in Boo et al. 2022). Of these, the only previous study on filled pauses in the speech of adults on the autism spectrum found a lower rate of filled pauses across lexical types (*uh* and *uhm*), while the remaining six studies considering children all report a lower proportion (or rate) of only *uhm*, but not *uh*, in the speech of autistic as compared to non-autistic participants.

These findings have led to a suggestion in some of the works cited above that the nasal filled pause type *uhm* might have a distinctly listener-oriented function, and that the pattern of a reduced production of *uhm*, specifically, might help to distinguish ASD from related diagnoses (Gorman et al. 2016) and serve as a pragmatic (Irvine et al. 2016) or even clinical marker (McGregor & Hadden 2020). Gorman et al. (2016) further suggest that "fillers (...) may be a useful target for intervention" (p. 862). Such speculations have to be treated with caution, however. Not only is the amount of evidence rather limited to date, especially when taking into account the serious and pertinent issue of publication bias (whereby studies that find a "significant" effect are vastly more likely to be published than those that do not; DeVito & Goldacre 2019, Easterbrook et al. 1991, John et al. 2012, Sterling 1959). More specifically, the relevant pattern of a reduced use of *uhm* (specifically and exclusively) does not seem to hold true for autistic adults, as suggested by the only relevant previous study (Lake et al. 2011) as well as the findings presented in this section.

5.4.1.2 Current study

With the current study, I aim to make a novel contribution to the literature on filled pause production in ASD by 1) analysing conversations between autistic adults (for the first time) and 2) considering the prosodic realisation of filled pauses in the context of ASD. As emphasised throughout this book, investigating the behaviour of disposition-matched dyads seems to me the most promising way to gain insights into what might justifiably be called an autistic conversation style (Bolis et al. 2017, Davis & Crompton 2021, Milton 2012, Mitchell et al. 2021, Sheppard et al. 2016). Furthermore, while there is a substantial amount of previous research on the prosodic realisation of filled pauses in the general population, this aspect has not been considered in work on ASD to date. Since previous findings point to a very clear cross-linguistic tendency for filled pauses being produced with flat or level intonation, the focus in this study lies mainly on investigating whether there is any deviation from this convention in the data set under investigation. Based on current knowledge and findings regarding the intonation of backchannels (§5.3), it can be speculated that the exact prosodic realisation of filled pauses may be similarly impactful.

5.4.2 Results

I will first present results on the rate and type of filled pauses, and then discuss prosodic aspects. The average duration of filled pauses was very similar across groups (ASD: 423 ms; CTR: 456 ms), with a grand mean of 444 ms (SD = 247), and will therefore not be considered in any more detail in the following.

5.4.2.1 Rate of filled pauses

Both groups produced an identical average rate of filled pauses per minute (3.63). Underlying this was a very high degree of by-dyad variability in both groups, with filled pause rates ranging from 0.82 to 4.82. Furthermore, it was found that interlocutors in the ASD group seemed to adapt less to each other within dyads compared to dyads in the CTR group. Specifically, the difference between by-speaker filled pause rates within dyads tended to be much lower in the CTR group (mean = 0.53; SD = 0.44) than in the ASD group (mean = 1.56; SD = 1.18), and ASD dyads also accounted for the four greatest within-dyad differences; see Figure 5.13.

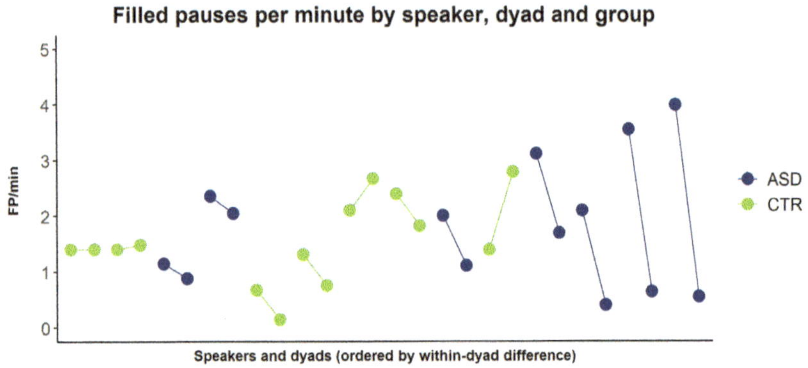

Figure 5.13: Rate of filled pauses produced per minute of dialogue, by speaker, dyad and group. Speakers within a dyad are connected by lines representing within-dyad differences (by which dyads are ordered on the x-axis). ASD group in blue, CTR group in green.

As for backchannels (see details in §5.3.2.1), Bayesian negative binomial regression modelling of rates by dyad was used to test the group difference. Model output unambiguously confirms that there was no difference in the rate of filled pauses between the ASD and the CTR group (mean δ = -0.4; 95% CI [-1.63, 0.78]; $P(\delta > 0) = 0.72$); see the accompanying repository for further details on the Bayesian model (https://osf.io/6zu4g/).

Looking at different stages of dialogue reveals an overall trend for both groups to produce more filled pauses in the later stages of dialogue. However, those differences were far from robust within and across groups due to massive dyad-specific variability, as confirmed by Bayesian modelling (see repository for details). Variability was greater in the ASD group than in the CTR group. The mean rate of filled pauses per minute across groups was 3.19 before resolution of the first Mismatch and 3.73 after resolution of the first Mismatch.

For speaker roles, proportions were calculated, i.e. the summed duration of filled pauses was divided by the summed duration of all speech for givers and followers separately, as opposed to a calculation of FP rates (as for backchannels; see §5.3.2.1). Proportions were calculated instead of rates because speaking times differed considerably between speaker roles.

There was a tendency across groups for instruction givers to produce a higher average proportion of filled pauses (3.71% overall) than instruction followers (2.41% overall). Bayesian modelling taking into account dyad as a random factor suggests that this difference between roles was reliable across groups (mean $\delta = 1.72$; 95% CI [-0.01, 3.61]; $P(\delta > 0) = 0.95$). Within groups, however, the difference between roles was shown to be reliable only for the ASD group ($P(\delta > 0) = 0.95$) and not for the CTR group ($P(\delta > 0) = 0.84$). This discrepancy seems to stem from a higher degree of dyad-specific variability in the CTR group. Overall, the behaviour of 9 out of 14 dyads clearly reflected the group level pattern of more and/or longer filled pauses produced by instruction givers.

5.4.2.2 Lexical choice: *uh* vs. *uhm*

There is a long tradition in the literature on filled pauses of contrasting and comparing nasal (*uhm*) with non-nasal (*uh*) filled pauses. I followed this in dividing all filled pauses into these two categories (see §5.2). In all the following analyses, I will use *uh* to refer to filled pauses without a final nasal and *uhm* to refer to filled pauses with a final nasal. I use this transcription to ensure consistency and comparability with previous studies (on languages other than German), even though filled pauses are almost always represented orthographically as <äh(m)> in German language materials.

Choice of filled pause type was very similar at the group level. Both groups used more *uhm* than *uh* overall, although this preference was slightly stronger for the CTR group (60% *uhm*) than for the ASD group (55.3% *uhm*). This group pattern obscures a very high degree of individual variability, however, with *uhm* proportions ranging from 0% to 100% for different speakers; see Figure 5.14. Although fewer CTR speakers showed a preference for *uhm* (7 out of 14) than ASD speakers did (11 out of 14), the preference for one filled pause type over another was not systematic at the group level and instead seems to be a correlate of individual variability.

This high degree of individual specificity combined with the very small initial difference of group averages makes it unsurprising that Bayesian regression modelling of *uhm* proportions by speaker strongly suggests that there was no reliable group difference in choice of filled pause type (mean $\delta = -4.9$; 95% CI [-15.78, 6.08]; $P(\delta > 0) = 0.77$; further details in the accompanying files).

5.4.2.3 Intonational realisation

For the prosodic analysis, 176 tokens were discarded because pitch information was not available or was found to be unreliable upon manual inspection (e.g. be-

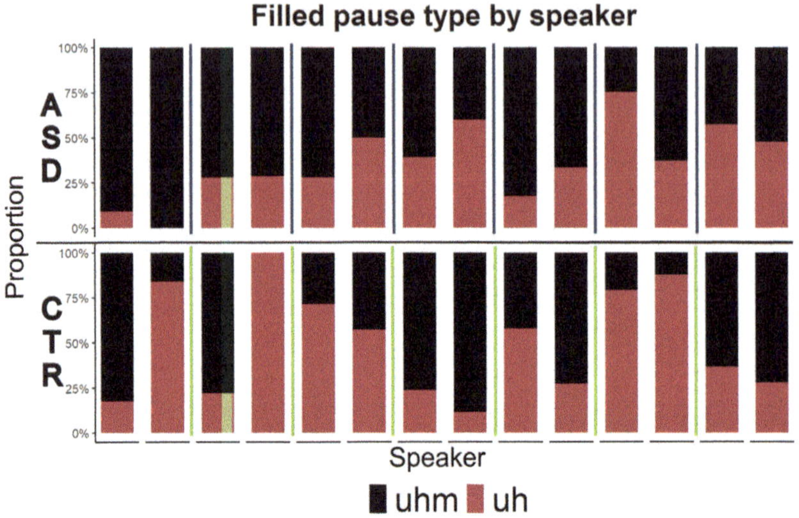

Figure 5.14: Proportion of filled pause type by group and speaker (as a percentage of their total filled pause productions). *Uhm* (nasal) in black, *uh* (non-nasal) in pink. ASD group in the top row, CTR group in the bottom row. Speakers from the same dyad are plotted next to each other; dyads are separated by vertical lines.

cause tokens were extremely short and/or produced with non-modal voice quality). This left 851 of the original 1027 tokens (82.9%). Note that one speaker (M14, from the CTR group) did not produce any filled pause tokens suitable for prosodic analysis (having produced only 2 filled pauses in total; the average number of filled pauses produced per speaker is 37). Therefore, the following analyses will be limited to the remaining 27 speakers (14 ASD; 13 CTR).

Continuous analysis

A continuous analysis of intonation contours on filled pauses revealed very little difference between groups. Both groups produced average values very close to 0 ST, representing little to no pitch movement, i.e. level intonation contours. This is expected according to previous results on the intonational realisation of filled pauses. Mean values were slightly closer to 0 for the CTR group (mean = -0.29; SD = 1.26) compared to the ASD group (mean = -0.44; SD = 1.51). Bayesian modelling broadly confirms this trend, but also strongly suggests that it is unlikely to be a robust difference between groups (mean $\delta = 0.25$; 95% CI [-0.16, 0.67]; $P(\delta > 0) = 0.84$; further details in the accompanying files).

Categorical analysis

To better account for the special status of level contours (the typical realisation) in the intonation of filled pauses, a categorical analysis was conducted in which all filled pauses with pitch movement within the range ±1 ST were categorised as *level*. The tokens exceeding these values were categorised as rises (positive values) and falls (negative values), respectively (see §5.3.2.3 for details and rationale).

Across filled pause types, the CTR group produced a considerably higher proportion of the expected and widely attested level contours on filled pauses (70.3%) than the ASD group (55.3%), who produced higher proportions of both rises and falls instead; see Figure 5.15. Falling intonation was the second most common realisation in both groups, with rising intonation the least frequent.

Proportion of level contours by speaker was used as the dependent variable for Bayesian modelling. The model output confirms that the group difference in prosodic realisation is robust (mean δ = 12.99; 95% CI [4.28, 21.87]; $P(\delta > 0)$ = 0.99; further details in the accompanying files).

Speaker-specific analysis confirms this pattern in showing, for instance, that 9 out of the 10 lowest proportions of level contours were produced by autistic speakers, whereas the 5 highest proportions of level contours were produced by non-autistic speakers (range 23.1% – 90%; see Figure C.2 in Appendix C).

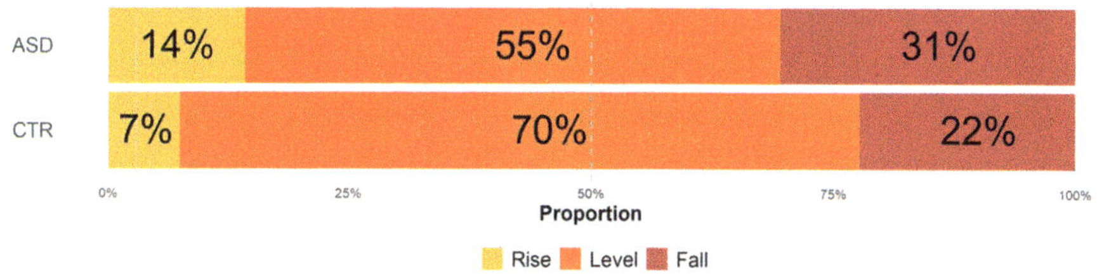

Figure 5.15: Intonation contour by group. Rising contours in yellow, level contours in orange and falling contours in red. Level contours were defined as all tokens with a pitch difference in the range ±1 semitone.

Comparing the two filled pause types *uh* and uhm across groups, it was found that *uh* was more often produced with the canonical level contour (70%) than *uhm* (62.1%). Bayesian modelling of the proportions of level contours by filled pause type (*uhm* was the reference level) and speaker (which was treated as a random factor) confirms this as a robust difference (mean $\delta = 17.05$; 95% CI [9.23, 24.82]; $P(\delta > 0) = 1$).

Table 5.3 shows the proportions of level contours used by group and filled pause type. It is clear that level contours constituted the preferred intonational realisation of filled pauses across groups and types (followed by falls, and then rises, which were only rarely used). The pattern is comparatively less obvious for productions by autistic speakers, however. The ASD group produced fewer level contours than the CTR group for both *uhm* and *uh*, but the difference between groups is clearer for *uhm*, as only 49.5% of tokens in the ASD group were produced with a level contour, compared to 68.9% in the CTR group. However, a high degree of by-speaker variability underlies these group-level results and hence, there is no clear effect of the interaction of lexical type and intonation contour in a group-level comparison.

Table 5.3: Proportion of intonation contour by group and filled pause type (level proportions in bold).

Group	Type	Contour	Proportion
ASD	uhm	Fall	32.61%
ASD	**uhm**	**Level**	**49.46%**
ASD	uhm	Rise	17.93%
ASD	uh	Fall	27.03%
ASD	**uh**	**Level**	**64.86%**
ASD	uh	Rise	8.11%
CTR	uhm	Fall	22.09%
CTR	**uhm**	**Level**	**68.90%**
CTR	uhm	Rise	9.01%
CTR	uh	Fall	22.64%
CTR	**uh**	**Level**	**72.64%**
CTR	uh	Rise	4.72%

A Bayesian model of proportion of intonation contour by speaker, including the interaction between group and filled pause type and with speaker as a random effect, provides conclusive evidence that 1) fewer level contours were produced by autistic speakers than controls for both *uh* (mean $\delta = -14.28$; 95% CI [−25.91, −1.51]; $P(\delta > 0) = 0.96$) and *uhm* (mean $\delta = -10$; 95% CI [−19.75, 0.32]; $P(\delta > 0) = 0.95$) and 2) that *uh* was produced with a higher proportion of level contours than *uhm* in both the ASD group (mean $\delta = 16.52$; 95% CI [6.47, 26.12]; $P(\delta > 0) = 1$) and the CTR group (mean $\delta = 20.8$; 95% CI [9.8, 31.45]; $P(\delta > 0) = 1$). Although the difference between groups for intonational realisation was slightly greater for *uhm* compared to *uh*, there is no robust effect for the interaction between group and filled pause type (mean $\delta = 4.29$; 95% CI [-9.26, 17.84]; $P(\delta > 0) = 0.71$).

Diversity of prosodic realisation (entropy)

As in the analysis of backchannels (Section 5.3.2.3), Shannon entropy (H) was used as a measure of diversity in order to quantify proportional differences. In the case of the prosodic realisation of filled pauses, higher entropy values are indicative of more unusual behaviour, as speakers were expected to produce a (very) large proportion of filled pauses with a single intonational contour (level). More predictable and less diverse behaviour is represented with lower entropy values ($H = 0$ if only one contour was used for all tokens). Based on the results described above, we can expect to find higher entropy values for autistic speakers (as they produced fewer level contours). The highest possible entropy value in this case is 1.58 (equal proportions for all three types of rises).

Results at the group level indeed reveal a higher entropy value for the ASD group (1.4) compared to the CTR group (1.12). Speaker-specific analysis confirms this pattern as, e.g., six out of the seven highest entropy values were recorded for autistic speakers; see Figure 5.16.

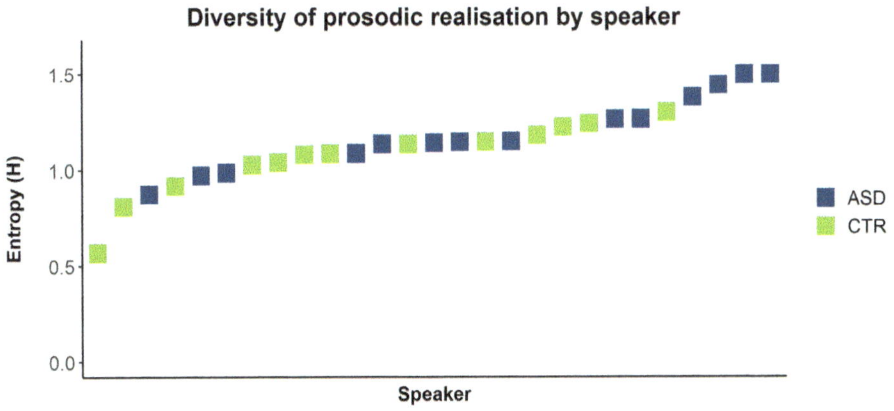

Figure 5.16: Entropy as a diversity measure of the prosodic realisation (rising, level or falling) of filled pauses, by speaker. Higher entropy values (H; on the y-axis) represent a more diverse realisation. ASD group in blue, CTR group in green.

Bayesian modelling of entropy values by speaker confirms the group-level difference in the intonational realisation of filled pauses as a robust effect (mean $\delta = -0.14$; 95% CI [-0.28, 0]; $P(\delta > 0) = 0.96$).

It has to be noted that entropy operationalised this way does not specifically measure proportions of level contours (as in the preceding section), but rather the diversity of intonation contours used. This means that if a speaker (unusually and unexpectedly) showed a clear preference for a non-level intonation contour (rise or fall), this behaviour would still be represented by a low entropy value. Indeed, 5 out of the 28 speakers in the data set under investigation did show a preference for falling instead of level contours in the realisation of filled pauses. However, especially as four out of those five speakers were part of the ASD group, this does not mitigate the fact that separate but related evidence has been presented for the observations 1) that autistic speakers produced fewer filled pauses with the canonical level contour and 2) that autistic speakers were more diverse in the intonational realisation of filled pauses.

5.4.3 Summary

The results presented in this section show that autistic and non-autistic speakers did not differ (at all) in the rate of filled pauses produced, nor in their preference of filled pause type (both preferring *uhm* over *uh*). The only group-level difference was in prosodic realisation, with ASD speakers producing fewer filled pauses realised with the typical level intonation contour than CTR speakers (although both groups did show a preference for level contours overall). Additionally, interlocutors in the CTR group seemed to adapt more to each other in terms of the rate of filled pauses produced compared to the ASD group. It is also interesting to note that the more frequent lexical type *uhm* was less consistently produced with a level contour, across groups, although this could simply be related to the fact that *uhm* was, on average, almost twice as long as *uh*. This increase in duration might in itself have led to the production of more falling contours (see §5.5 and Fuchs et al. 2015, Gussenhoven & Rietveld 1988).

5.5 Silent pauses

To complement the analysis of filled pauses (and the analysis of silent gaps between turns in Chapter 4), an analysis of silent pauses (within speaker-turns) was conducted.

5.5.1 Background

Silent pauses feature in the majority of spoken utterances, and they are particularly prevalent in conversational speech. While there is a solid amount of general research on the topic, and in the context of second-language speech in particular (Bradlow et al. 2017, De Jong & Bosker 2013), very little is known about the use of silent pauses in atypical populations, such as in the speech of persons diagnosed with ASD.

Previous work on silent pause use in ASD seems to be limited to three studies comparing autistic speakers with matched controls, with contradictory results. In Thurber & Tager-Flusberg (1993), fewer silent pauses in picture book narrations by English-speaking autistic children are reported. In contrast, Lake et al. (2011) report a higher rate of silent pauses in interview-style conversations between experimenters and English-speaking autistic adults. Finally, Engelhardt et al. (2017) found equivalent silent pause rates for autistic and matched non-autistic adults in a sentence repetition task.

Crucial differences in the age of participants and/or speech material make comparison with the corpus under investigation difficult in the cases of Thurber & Tager-Flusberg (1993), Engelhardt et al. (2017). As these confounding factors are less of a concern regarding the work by Lake et al. (2011) (age range and speech data being similar to the data at hand), I will focus on this latter study for comparison.

Lake et al. (2011) report a higher rate of silent pauses in autistic adults compared to non-autistic controls, but did not examine any silent pauses with a duration of under 2 seconds. The authors provide no specific reasons for using this extremely high cut-off point, only stating that "this was done in order to ensure that we excluded normal prosodic pauses" (p. 138). The sheer utility of such a threshold can further be called into question from a pragmatic–analytic point of view, as employing it entails excluding almost all silent pauses in a given data set: speakers from the control group in Lake et al. (2011) in fact did not produce any silent pauses longer than 2 seconds.

For this study, separate analyses were conducted of 1) silent pauses of any duration, 2) a subset of silent pauses over 2 seconds in duration (for comparison with Lake et al. 2011) and 3) silent pauses of 700 ms or longer, a subset of 1) and a superset of 2) (see §5.5.3.3 for rationale).

In addition to simply comparing the rate and duration of silent pauses, other potential group differences were explored in the form of the distributional characteristics of silent pauses. Specifically, it was examined which effect the lexical form of a preceding filled pause (*uh* or *uhm*) had on the duration of the following silent pause. This is chiefly inspired by the highly influential work in Clark & Fox Tree (2002) comparing the use of *uh* and *uhm* in spontaneous speech. The authors claim that there is a considerable difference in the average duration of silences following *uh* as compared to *uhm*, with *uhm* preceding silences of at least twice the duration of silences following *uh*. In a comparison of autistic and non-autistic children, Lunsford et al. (2010) confirmed this effect for their CTR, but not their ASD group.

While Clark & Fox Tree (2002) also showed, in a binary distinction, that silences following "lengthened" productions of both *uh* and *uhm* were considerably longer overall, the duration of the *uh* vs. *uhm* tokens themselves was not controlled for. In fact, to my knowledge, none of the subsequent papers examining this phenomenon involved an analysis that systematically controlled for the inherent average duration of *uh* and *uhm*.

This is a serious concern since, in the current data set at least, *uhm* is considerably longer (521 ms) than *uh* (329 ms) on average. Thus, it is important to establish whether and to what extent the effect ascribed to a difference in filled pause type (nasal vs. non-nasal) is in fact simply due to filled pause duration, independent of whether a final nasal was present (which for simple reasons of physiology and aerodynamics increases the likelihood of longer durations). An attempt was thus made to replicate the relevant effect while controlling for the confound of filled pause duration, all in the context of investigating differences between the ASD and CTR group in the current data set.

5.5.2 Data

The corpus contains a total of 3473 silent pauses. Portions of dialogue that contained only audible breathing, clicks, and similar noises were counted as being part of silent intervals. In contrast, all other speech sounds, including filled pauses, were counted as being part of IPUs. While it has to be acknowledged that most such "silent" pauses are not completely silent from a strictly acoustic perspective (Belz & Trouvain 2019), I chose to adhere to the conventional definition outlined above, since the main aim of this study is to enable comparison with the (sparse) previous literature on silent pauses in ASD as well as with the more general literature on the topic.

For the analysis of silences following filled pauses, all 1027 filled pause tokens in the data set as well as their surrounding linguistic context (see §5.4) were investigated. If filled pauses were followed not by any period of silence, but instead directly by another utterance (by either of the interlocutors), a duration of 0 was assigned to the following silence. All relevant code, scripts, model specifications and data frames are available in the *OSF* repository at https://osf.io/bph2t/.

5.5.3 Results

I will report results first on silent pause rate, using different durational cut-offs, and then on silences following *uh* vs. *uhm*.

5.5.3.1 All silent pause tokens

The mean duration of silent pauses was close to identical across groups, with means of 677 ms (SD = 563) for the ASD and 628 ms (SD = 527) for the CTR group. The mean rate of silent pauses was exactly identical across groups, with a value of 12.2 silent pauses per minute. A dyad-specific analysis of silent-pause rates also gives no indications of ASD-specific behaviour; see Figure 5.17. Note that there was a considerable degree of by-dyad variability and overlap between groups, not only for this analysis, but also all the ones described below.

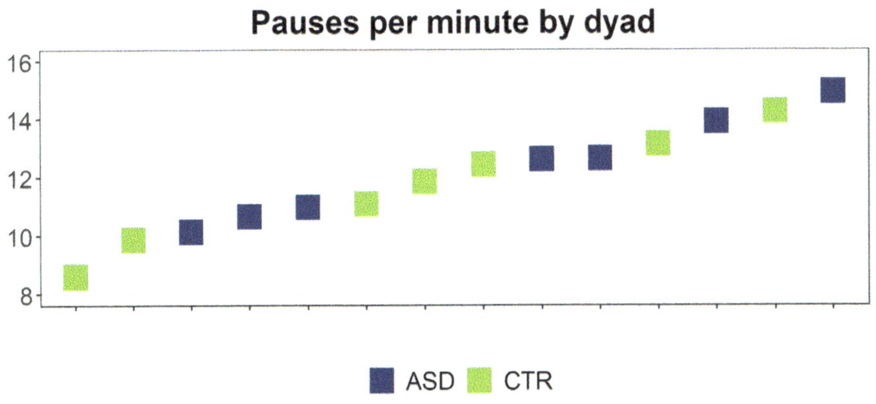

Figure 5.17: Rate of silent pauses by dyad and group (ASD in blue, CTR in green).

5.5.3.2 Silent pauses >2 seconds

To allow for a direct comparison with Lake et al. (2011), a subset of all silent pauses with a duration of over 2 seconds was analysed. Silent pauses of this kind were very rare in the corpus under investigation (73 tokens, or 2%, of the total 3473). The number of such pauses produced by each dyad ranged from 0 to 13.

The ASD group produced a higher mean rate of long silent pauses (>2 s) per minute (0.33; n = 34) than the CTR group (0.21; n = 39); see Figure 5.18. Given the low overall number of instances, a more intuitive way of stating the same observation is that a 20-minute dialogue (average duration) would typically contain seven long pauses (>2 s) in the ASD group and four long pauses (>2 s) in the CTR group.

Bayesian Poisson regression suggests that this was a robust difference between groups (mean δ = -0.12; 95% CI [-0.23, -0.01]; $P(\delta > 0)$ = 0.97). However, the proximity of the higher end of the credible interval to zero and the very low overall number of observations are reasons for exercising some caution in the interpretation of these data.

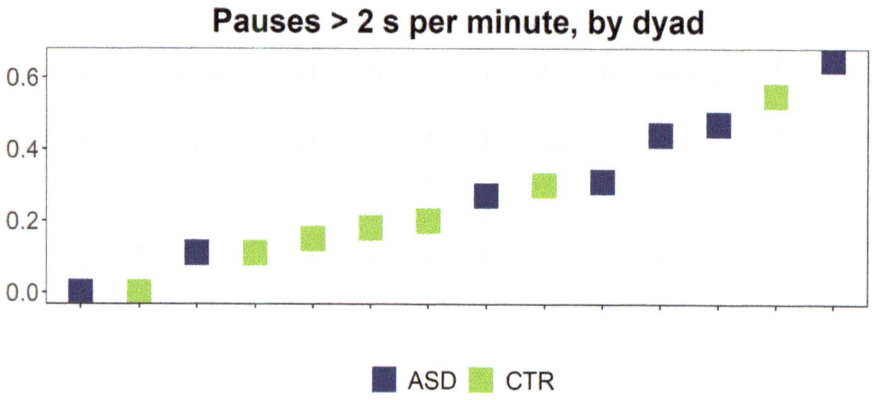

Figure 5.18: Rate of silent pauses >2 s in duration, by dyad and group (ASD in blue, CTR in green).

5.5.3.3 Silent pauses ≥700 milliseconds

For a more reliable and representative metric of long pauses in dialogue, a lower cut-off value, at 700 milliseconds, was used. This particular threshold was chosen mainly because it clearly exceeds mean pause durations in the data set used here (646 ms across groups) as well as in previous work (De Jong & Bosker 2013, Cho & Hirst 2006, Megyesi & Gustafson-Capková 2002). The same value was used for categorising long silent gaps between speakers (in §4.4.2), based on the finding that gaps of 700 ms or longer are perceived as unusual by listeners and often cue repair initiations or non-affiliating responses (Kendrick 2015, Kendrick & Torreira 2015, Roberts & Francis 2013). As the difference between within-speaker pauses and between-speaker gaps structurally lies only in who takes the following turn, the relevant findings further support the use of a 700-millisecond threshold for silent pauses.

Using this cut-off point leaves far more observations for analysis (n = 1052) and will therefore also yield more robust and reliable results.

The group rate of silent pauses ≥700 ms was higher for the ASD group (4.02) than for the CTR group (3.52); see Figure 5.19. Although this group difference is not very large, Bayesian negative binomial regression shows the effect to be robust, confirming that the CTR group produced a lower rate of long silent pauses (≥700 ms) than the ASD group (mean δ = -0.5; 95% CI [-0.9, -0.1]; $P(\delta > 0) = 0.98$).

Thus, we can conclude that autistic dyads produced more long silent pauses than non-autistic dyads, independently of the exact cut-off point used to define a long pause, although no difference between groups was found when tokens of any duration were taken into account.

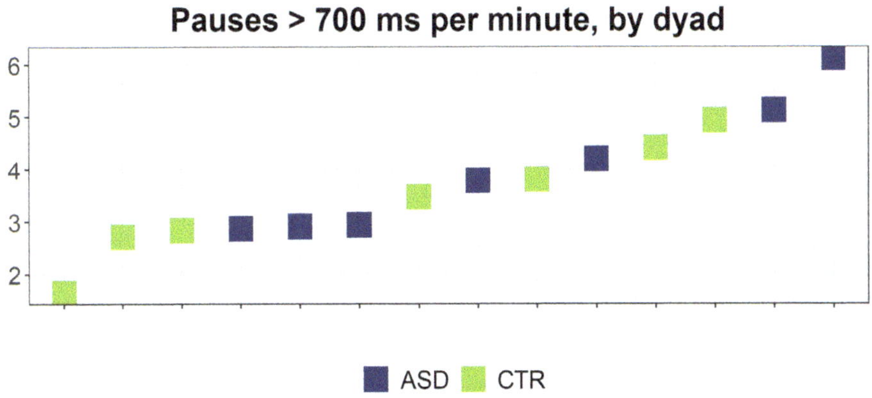

Figure 5.19: Rate of silent pauses ≥700 ms in duration, by dyad and group (ASD in blue, CTR in green).

5.5.3.4 Silence following *uh* vs. *uhm*

The effect of *uh* and *uhm* on subsequent stretches of silence was equivalent for the ASD and the CTR group overall, as *uhm* was followed by longer silences in both groups and for all analyses. I will therefore report results across groups below.

When disregarding filled pause duration (as in previous studies), a clear difference in the mean duration of following silence according to filled pause type was found: silences were on average 355 ms longer following *uhm* (mean = 541; SD = 1056) than following *uh* (mean = 186; SD = 517). Further, the proportion of filled pauses followed by a period of silence with a duration > 0 (i.e. not followed directly by speech) was calculated. This was the case more frequently for *uhm* (69.4%) than for *uh* (45%).

As a sanity check, a Bayesian linear regression model with a hurdle log-normal distribution was run to check whether filled pause duration, independent of filled pause type, could actually be shown to be correlated with the duration of the following silence at all. The model output unambiguously confirms this to be the case (mean $\delta = 0.29$; 95% CI [0.16, 0.43]; $P(\delta > 0) = 1$): longer filled pauses clearly tended to be followed by longer intervals of silence.

To conclusively establish whether differences between filled pause types were independent of the fact that *uhm* tokens in themselves were typically considerably longer than *uh* tokens, a model with log-normal distribution was fitted to the duration of the following silence, with speaker and, crucially, duration of filled pause, as random factors.

Results show that silences following *uhm* were indeed longer than those following *uh*, regardless of the duration of filled pause tokens, even though the difference was quite small (150 ms). More details on statistical modelling are reported below.

In the main model, only observations where filled pauses were followed by at least 200 ms of silence (i.e. followed by a new, separate IPU) were included. The difference between types is presented with *uhm* as the reference level. The model output shows the difference to be robust, even though the upper bound of the credible interval is close to zero (mean $\delta = -0.15$; 95% CI [-0.28, -0.02]; $P(\delta > 0) = 0.97$). A second model, including also all cases where the following silence was 0 (using a hurdle log-normal model), confirms the finding in also showing a robust effect for the difference between filled pause types (mean $\delta = -0.12$; 95% CI [-0.19, -0.07]; $P(\delta > 0) = 1$).

5.5.4 Summary

The analyses presented in this section show that there were more long silent pauses in conversations between autistic dyads as compared to non-autistic control dyads. This is broadly in line with results from one of the three previously published studies on the same topic (Lake et al. 2011), but stands in contradiction to an earlier account (Thurber & Tager-Flusberg 1993). No group differences were found when considering all silent pauses regardless of duration, nor for mean pause duration (similarly to results in Engelhardt et al. 2017). There was also no between-group difference regarding the effect of preceding filled pause type on subsequent silent pause duration. This stands in contrast to results in Lunsford et al. (2010), where longer silences following *uhm* were found for non-autistic, but not autistic children.

5.6 Laughter

While an analysis of laughter is not directly related to that of filled pauses (or related discourse markers such as backchannels), there are two reasons for including a preliminary analysis of rates of laughter here. First, laughter by a single speaker (rather than two speakers at once) often falls into the category of *non-Duchenne laughter* (Gervais & Wilson 2005, Keltner & Bonanno 1997, Mehu 2011), that is, it is used not to express genuine joy or amusement as a reaction to an outside stimulus, but rather it is self-generated and essentially emotionless. This kind of laughter can be observed in moments of nervousness or hesitation, among others (Pietrowicz et al. 2019, Ruch & Ekman 2001). Thus, laughter by a single speaker can be considered to at least sometimes be functionally related to filled pauses such as *uh* or *uhm*. Previous research suggests that individual laughter differs from shared (or overlapping) laughter in both form and function (Trouvain & Truong 2012, 2013, 2017, Truong & Trouvain 2012). Intriguingly, shared laughter seems to also be correlated with accommodation and convergence in a way that individual laughter is not.

Second, in discussions of the corpus and related results as well as in annotation and analysis of the data itself, it was anecdotally observed that autistic conversations seemed to contain far less laughter. This can also be related to the observations that Map Tasks tended to be completed in a much shorter amount of time in the ASD group and that autistic dyads produced fewer backchannels, in the sense that these patterns might reflect a more goal-oriented or functionally efficient way of navigating the task and the social interaction in itself.

The literature on laughter in ASD is very limited and characterised by inconclusive results, highlighting mainly a high degree of individual variability (Hudenko et al. 2009, Reddy et al. 2002) – indeed, essentially the same can be said about research on the frequency of laughter in non-autistic conversation (Trouvain & Truong 2017, Vettin & Todt 2004).

For pragmatic reasons, this account is limited to a superficial analysis of rates of laughter, leaving in-depth acoustic, prosodic and contextual analysis for future work. All instances of laughter in the corpus were annotated, counted, and labelled as being either individual laughter or shared (overlapping) laughter by both interlocutors within a dyad. Any instances where laughter from both speakers overlapped for at least 200 milliseconds were counted as shared laughter.

The corpus under investigation contains 385 bouts of laughter in total. A descriptive analysis at the group level reveals a clear tendency for higher rates of laughter in the CTR group compared to the ASD group, for both individual laughter (ASD: 0.67; CTR: 1.38) and shared laughter (ASD: 0.12; CTR: 0.29); see Figure 5.20. In other words, non-autistic dyads produced more than twice as much individual and shared laughter than autistic dyads on average. This pattern is supported by analysis at the dyad level. Strikingly, two out of seven ASD dyads did not produce any laughter whatsoever, whereas this was not the case for any CTR dyads, who also produced five out of the six highest overall rates of laughter (across types).

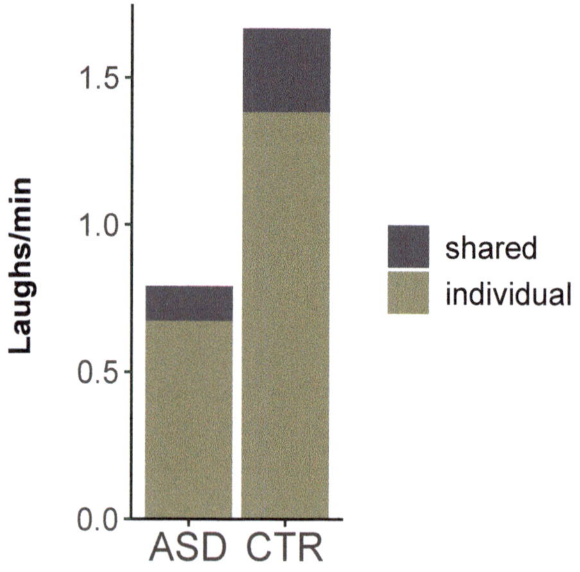

Figure 5.20: Rate of laughter per minute (y-axis) by group (x-axis) and type (shared / individual).

Bayesian negative binomial regression was used to analyse rates of individual and shared laughter per minute, as for the rates of backchannels (§5.3.2.1) and filled pauses (§5.4.2.1). Output from Bayesian modelling confirms the pattern described above in showing higher mean rates in CTR dyads for both individual laughter (mean δ = 1.09; 95% CI [0.02, 2.68]; $P(\delta > 0) = 0.95$) and shared laughter (mean δ = 0.25; 95% CI [0, 0.62]; $P(\delta > 0) = 0.95$). Although these trends are very strong, the lower ends of both credible intervals are (virtually) at zero, suggesting that observing no difference in laughter rate between groups would be not entirely incompatible with the model, the data and prior assumptions.

Due to the shortage of previous studies, it is not clear whether simply counting the number of bouts of laughter, independent of their duration and other characteristics, is the best shorthand for characterising laughter behaviour, even in a first exploratory analysis such as this one. To complement the analysis of laughter rates described above, *proportions* of laughter relative to dialogue duration were therefore also calculated. To do so, the duration of all instances of laughter (separately for individual laughter and shared laughter) produced within a dyad was summed, and this number was divided by the total duration of the respective conversation. Bouts of laughter are usually both relatively short (mean = 683 ms) and relatively rare (total combined duration of all tokens in the corpus = 263 seconds (~4 minutes) in a corpus with a total duration of 17065 seconds (~5 hours)). As a result, proportion values on a percent scale are very low (ranging from 0 to 0.0311). For ease of computation and analysis, these values were multiplied by 1000, resulting in *per cent mille* (pcm) values, ranging from 0 to 31.1.

Overall, the pattern of results found using the variable of laughter proportion very closely resembles that of results using the variable of laughter rates, thereby strengthening the validity of both measures. Higher laughter proportions were found for the CTR group in terms of both individual laughter (ASD: 7.78 pcm; CTR: 16 pcm) and shared laughter (ASD: 1.77 pcm; CTR: 2.68 pcm). Results are shown by dyad and laughter type in Figure 5.21.

There was substantial overlap across and considerable variability within groups. The differences between groups were less pronounced for proportions than they were for rates, especially in the case of shared laughter (which was rare across groups and dyads). Accordingly, Bayesian modelling of laughter proportion by dyad confirmed the observed group difference for individual laughter (mean δ = 7.63; 95% CI [2.9, 12.27]; $P(\delta > 0) = 0.99$), as it had done for rate of laughter, but not for shared laughter (mean δ = 1.45; 95% CI [-3.55, 6.59]; $P(\delta > 0) = 0.69$), in contrast to the analysis of laughter rates.

In sum, the ASD group produced considerably less laughter overall than the CTR group. This finding is robust – and independent of measurement (rate or proportion of laughter) – for individual laughter, but less clear for shared laughter.

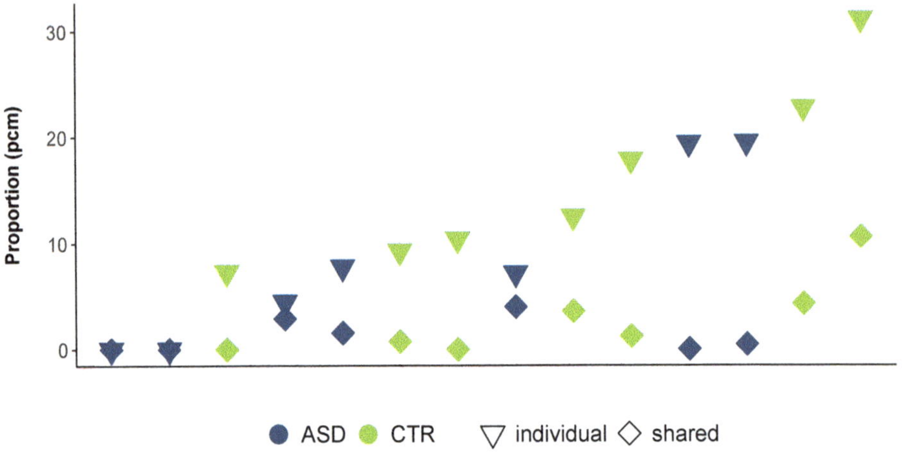

Figure 5.21: Proportion of laughter in pcm (*per cent mille*; y-axis) by group and dyad (x-axis). ASD group in blue, CTR group in green. Individual laughter represented with inverted triangles, shared laughter represented with diamonds. Dyads are ordered by combined proportion of individual and shared laughter.

5.7 Discussion

This chapter discussed the use of backchannels and filled pauses (as well as silent pauses and laughter) in German adults with and without a diagnosis of autism spectrum disorder. This is the first study of backchannels and of filled pauses in conversations between autistic adults.

In the corpus of semi-spontaneous speech under investigation, consistent differences in the rate as well as the lexical and intonational realisation of backchannels in the ASD group were found. Filled pauses differed between groups only in their prosodic realisation. Further, differences between groups were found for the frequency of silent pauses and, in a preliminary investigation, for laughter.

In this section, I will first interpret these results in some more detail and then point out the limitations of the current approach and the resulting potential for future work.

5.7.1 Backchannels: Reduced rate and flexibility in ASD

The result that autistic speakers produced fewer backchannels per minute than matched controls suggests that autistic individuals are overall less inclined to explicitly (and verbally) support the ongoing turn of their interlocutor. Backchannelling is a prosocial and specifically listener-oriented signal, which, moreover, is not governed by explicit rules and rather seems to follow complex, implicit, culture-specific conventions. Autistic individuals have been reported to show differences in understanding and interacting with their conversational partners. Furthermore, communication styles in ASD have been claimed to differ more from those of their non-autistic peers regarding implicit, rather than explicit, aspects of language. Thus, the analysis of backchannel rates can be linked to more general aspects of ASD.

The fact that there was a greater difference in the rate of backchannels between groups in the early stages compared with the remainder of the dialogue furthermore suggests that ASD dyads eventually produced a backchannelling style quite similar to that of CTR dyads, but that they took a certain amount of time to reach this point (reflecting results from the domain of turn-timing; see Chapter 4). It can further be speculated that a lower rate of BCs in the ASD group might indicate that autistic speakers focussed more on the collaborative completion of the task at hand, rather than on purely affiliative aspects of social interaction. This interpretation is supported by results from Dideriksen et al. (2019), who found that (non-autistic) speakers produced a higher rate of BCs in fully free conversations compared with task-oriented conversations (such as Map Tasks; see also Janz 2022).

This observation can also be related to the fact that CTR dyads tended to take far longer to complete the task (mean duration: 26 minutes) than ASD dyads (mean duration: 15 minutes; see §4.4.4.2). Qualitative assessment clearly confirms that this increased duration was usually not due to greater difficulties with completing the task, but rather due to more conversational content of a purely social nature (essentially *small talk*). This is mirrored by a higher rate of laughter in the CTR group (as shown in §5.6) compared to the ASD group. These observations in themselves can be taken, if somewhat speculatively, as further support for the notion that ASD dyads were focussed more on efficient completion of the experimental task and less on purely social aspects of the interaction.

Backchannel productions in the ASD group were also characterised by a less flexible realisation regarding lexical choice. Autistic speakers tended to use a smaller range of different BC types, and in turn often showed a clear preference for one particular lexical type which was used for the majority of tokens. This is analogous to the findings for prosodic realisation: many autistic speakers predominantly used rises, across different BC types, whereas non-autistic speakers tended to show a more complex probabilistic mapping of different (proportions of) intonation contours to different types of backchannel. This pattern held true for all BC types except non-lexical *mmhm*, which was produced with rises in almost all cases by almost all speakers. I will further discuss the special status of *mmhm* and its relation to filled pauses below in §5.7.3.

Differences between groups aside, the current findings on the prosodic realisation of backchannels are significant in themselves, as earlier accounts (of backchannels in West Germanic languages) instead tended to assume a kind of 'default' BC contour (rising) for all different types of BCs. It is interesting to note that the prosodic realisation of the non-lexical BC *mmhm* comes closest to such a simple mapping – perhaps because its meaning has to be conveyed purely by means of prosody – and in turn particularly intriguing that many autistic speakers seemed to apply this one-to-one mapping to all different lexical types of BCs (in contrast to non-autistic speakers). This result can also be related to an earlier finding (involving speech from some of the same autistic subjects) according to which the ASD group showed a stronger preference (compared with a control group) for using one particular pitch accent type (H*) over other types (Krüger et al. 2018).

In sum, the findings reported suggest that a lower rate and a less variable realisation characterise backchannel production in ASD. We can conclude 1) that autistic speakers are less inclined to use BCs in order to support the ongoing turn of their interlocutor in the early stages of a social interaction and 2) that when they do so, productions are less diverse and less flexible. This latter observation can be seen as a specific, micro-level instantiation of the pattern of circumscribed and stereotypical behaviour that is used as a key diagnostic criterion for ASD at the macro level.

While this work is the first study of backchannelling in (semi-)spontaneous conversations between autistic adults, the finding that autistic dyads used fewer BCs is in line with results from the only two related studies published to date (Rifai et al. 2022, Yoshimura et al. 2020). In expanding our perspective beyond ASD, we can further compare the current findings to the extensive literature on BC productions across different cultures. This body of work suggests that listeners are highly sensitive to deviations from a given "standard" realisation of BCs and that they judge such deviations negatively. It thus stands to reason that the differences in backchanneling behaviour found in the ASD group in the current work might also lead to misunderstandings and negative impressions, at least in interactions with non-autistic interlocutors. I would nevertheless like to stress once again that while a comparative analysis of cross-cultural communication on the one hand and autistic vs. non-autistic communication on the other hand doubtlessly has a certain heuristic value and intuitive appeal, cultural differences are obviously not equivalent to differences in cognitive style, regardless of phenotypical similarities in certain aspects of social interaction.

5.7.2 Filled pauses: Differences specifically in prosodic realisation

It was shown that autistic and non-autistic speakers did not differ (at all) in the rate of filled pauses produced, nor in their preference of filled pause type (both preferring *uhm* over *uh*). The only group-level difference detected concerns the prosodic realisation of filled pauses, with ASD speakers producing fewer FPs with the typical level intonation contour than CTR speakers (although both groups did show a preference for level contours overall). Additionally, interlocutors in the CTR group seemed to adapt more to each other in terms of the rate of filled pauses produced compared to the ASD group. It is also interesting to note that the more frequent lexical type *uhm* was less consistently produced with a level contour, across groups, although this could simply be related to the fact that *uhm* was, on average, almost twice as long as *uh*. This increase in duration might in itself have led to the production of more falling contours.

While the study reported here is the first to analyse prosodic aspects of filled pause production in ASD, we can compare the current results on rate and lexical choice with previous studies on these aspects. Superficially, the fact that no differences were found in filled pause rate or preference of type (*uhm* over *uh*) perhaps surprisingly supports the findings from only one study (Suh et al. 2014) and stands in contrast to the other relevant findings (Gorman et al. 2016, Irvine et al. 2016, Jones et al. 2022, Lake et al. 2011, Lunsford et al. 2010, McGregor & Hadden 2020, Parish-Morris et al. 2017).

A direct comparison with the results reported here, however, is not possible as none of the previous studies investigated semi-structured conversations between autistic adults, instead tending to focus on speech elicited in more highly structured, formal contexts and produced by children (usually interacting with non-autistic adults). A related issue is the inclusion of (autistic and non-autistic) speaker groups with a very wide age range in previous work, leading to one such sample being described as "children from 8 to 21 years old" (Suh et al. 2014: p. 1684).

Findings from the only other study investigating filled pause productions by autistic adults (Lake et al. 2011) crucially differ from the findings reported here. No difference in filled pause rate was detected in the current analysis, whereas this earlier study found a lower rate for both *uh* and *uhm* in their ASD group. At the same time, there is an important similarity between this previous study and the current work, as in both cases there is no evidence for a special role of *uhm*, in particular, for distinguishing the behaviour of autistic and control subjects (in contrast to all the studies on autistic children mentioned above). While I do not wish to speculate widely about causes and implications on the basis of two studies, it does seem plausible 1) that the role of *uhm* as being more listener-oriented compared to *uh* may have been exaggerated in some previous research, at least where such conclusions were drawn on the basis of the fact that some autistic speakers seemed to produce *uhm* less often than control speakers, and 2) that continuous development and successful social camouflaging might play important roles in autistic adults behaving more similarly to their non-autistic peers than is the case for children.

More generally, as filled pauses are most prevalent and functionally important in conversational interaction (Corley & Hartsuiker 2003, Fox Tree 2001), the external validity of results based on speech elicited through, e.g., highly structured interviews with children (Gorman et al. 2016), picture story narrations (Suh et al. 2014) or descriptions of a series of paintings with the added task of simultaneously tapping an index finger as fast as possible (Irvine et al. 2016) has to be questioned. Speculations as to the pro-social nature of filled pauses are similarly problematic when they are founded on this kind of speech data. Engelhardt et al. (2017) rightly point out some important issues in the interpretation of conversational behaviours as being either speaker- or listener-oriented in such contexts (and also criticise the fact that previous research did not appropriately account for individual differences). Somewhat puzzlingly, the authors then proceed to describe production data from a sentence-repetition task, which did not yield a single filled pause token (as might be expected, partly because there is no need in this context to use filled pauses to facilitate the planning of an utterance).

To sum up, as the current analysis did not confirm previous finding of filled pauses being produced at a lower rate in ASD, or that nasal filled pauses (*uhm*) are dispreferred in ASD, it seems reasonable to call into question 1) the causal interpretation of filled pauses as specifically and exclusively "other-directed" signals (e.g. Lake et al. 2011) and 2) the appropriateness of using characteristics of filled pauses, specifically the production of *uhm*, as a pragmatic or clinical marker for ASD, as has been suggested in previous work (Irvine et al. 2016, McGregor & Hadden 2020). In general, the use of *uhm* might well differ from that of *uhm* in important and general ways. For instance, it has been shown that silences following *uhm* are longer than silences following *uh* (§5.5; Clark & Fox Tree 2002). However, just as no differences between the ASD and the CTR group were found in this regard here, both the results presented in the current work and in the previous study by Lake et al. (2011) suggest that while the use of *uhm* may differ between autistic and non-autistic children, this is not necessarily the case for adult speakers.

5.7.3 Comparing *mmhm* and *uhm*

I proposed in Section 5.4.1 that, functionally, backchannels and filled pauses are polar opposites, since backchannels are used by listeners to support the ongoing turn of the interlocutor, whereas filled pauses are used by speakers to hold the floor and retain their own turn. In other words, filled pauses are "the most common way to hold the turn" for a speaker, while backchannels are signals by the listener that they are "paying attention to the speaker and....encouraging him [sic]" (Ward 2019: pp. 157, 162). This can be related to the higher rates of backchannels but lower rates of filled pauses found in the speech of instruction followers compared to instruction givers in the current analysis.

With this in mind, consider that the most frequent type of filled pause in the corpus under investigation is *uhm* (n = 600) and the second most frequent type of backchannel is *mmhm* (n = 456). Thus, there are over 1000 cases in which these classes of discourse marker are extremely similar in segmental form (some tokens from both classes are indeed identically produced, as /m/), while having directly contrasting functions in dialogue management.

This brings us back to the observation that the non-lexical backchannel *mmhm* stands out among other BC types, as it was very consistently (in 90% of cases) produced with rising intonation. Compare this to the filled pause type *uhm*, which was produced with a rising contour in only 12% of all cases (typically produced with a level contour instead).

Relevant results from the continuous analysis of intonation contours are shown in Figure 5.22, confirming that there was very little overlap in the distributions of ST values for *mmhm* (mean = 5.87 ST) and *uhm* (mean = -0.33 ST). Another way to describe the same pattern would be to say that 88.4% of pitch values for *mmhm* exceeded the 95th percentile of pitch values for *uhm* (1.67 ST).

I propose that this complementary distribution of intonational realisation is not merely a reflection of the opposing functions of backchannels and filled pauses, but may be causally related to it. Following this hypothesis, speakers are (at least implicitly) aware of both the contrast in function and the similarity in segmental form between *mmhm* and *uhm* (and the absence of lexical meaning in both cases) and therefore use suprasegmental features (i.e. intonation) in order to distinguish between *mmhm* and *uhm* in order to ensure accurate transmission of their communicative intent. While it is true that the potential for misunderstanding is limited by the fact that *uhm* is usually (but not always) uttered by speakers (turn-holders) whereas *mmhm* is almost exclusively uttered by listeners, this does not negate the facts that 1) the similarities in segmental form remain a potential source of confusion, 2) listeners are highly sensitive to *any* deviances

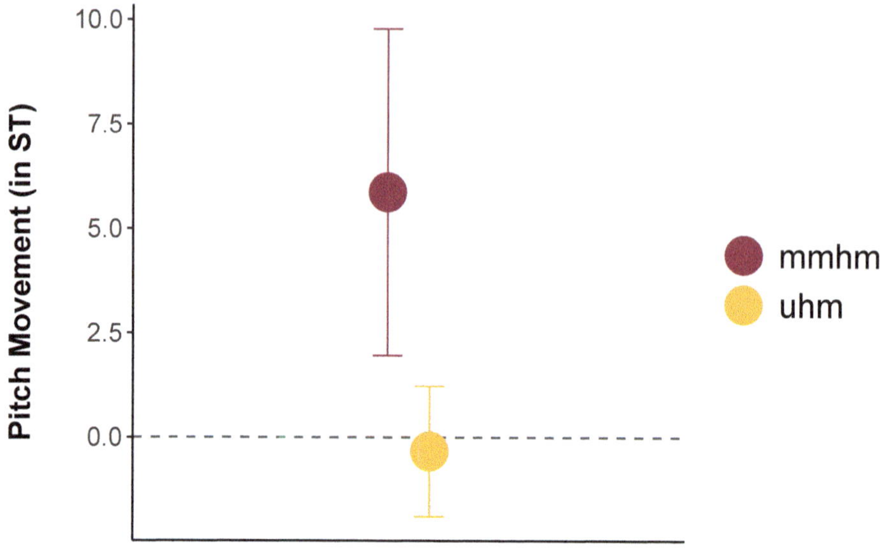

Figure 5.22: Mean values for pitch contours produced on the backchannel *mmhm* (in burgundy) and the filled pause *uhm* (in yellow), across groups. Error bars represent one standard deviation from the mean.

in the precise realisation of discourse markers and 3) redundancy of this kind is not an unusual feature of spoken communication in general (Winter 2014, Winter & Wedel 2016, Coretta et al. 2023, Aylett & Turk 2004).

In sum, I have suggested that the contrasting functions of filled pauses and backchannels are reflected in their prosodic realisation. Specifically, there is very little overlap in the intonation contours used for the segmentally similar backchannel type *mmhm* (typically rising) and the filled pause type *uhm* (typically level).

5.7.4 Silent pauses

In expanding the current investigation beyond backchannels and filled pauses (and silent gaps), evidence was presented for a robust tendency towards a higher rate of long silent pauses in conversations between autistic compared to non-autistic dyads, while at the same time many similarities in the silent pause use of both groups were found.

While differences were thus rather subtle overall, the higher rate of long silent pauses in the ASD group is still likely to have a discernible effect on spoken interaction (De Jong & Bosker 2013, Goldman-Eisler 1968), and might thus contribute to perceptions of a difference in communication styles. This is all the more true when considering that the current work provides evidence for idiosyncratic behaviour by the same autistic speakers in the related domain of turn-timing, where they produced more long silent gaps between speakers compared to non-autistic dyads (but only in the early stages of conversations; see Chapter 4).

Besides uncovering group differences in silent pause use, the current study replicates the finding that silences tend to be longer following *uhm* compared to *uh* (Clark & Fox Tree 2002). The analysis presented here does not merely provide a replication, however, but rather extends and qualifies the original finding, as the duration of filled pauses was added as a random factor in a Bayesian regression model. This way, it could explicitly be shown that the effect described is independent of intrinsic filled pause length (importantly, as *uhm* tends to be longer than *uh*).

Moreover, the current results suggest that the effect of longer silences following *uhm* compared to *uh* is more subtle than previously described. While a twofold difference in silence duration according to filled pause type is reported in Clark & Fox Tree (2002), a difference of only 150 ms (with an average silent pause duration of 646 ms) when factoring in filled pause duration was found in the analyses presented here. It is not obvious how relevant such a relatively small difference might be in real-life spoken interaction – this question will have to be left open here and is hoped to inform future perception experiments.

5.7.5 Limitations

There are a number of limitations to the approaches used here to analyse backchannels and filled pauses.

First, it has to be acknowledged that task-based rather than fully free conversations were investigated. The experimental setup also deliberately limited participants to the spoken modality by placing an opaque barrier between them during the Map Task experiment. There is little doubt that visual signals such as head nods, gesture and eye gaze can be used in ways that are functionally equivalent to spoken backchannels (Bevacqua et al. 2010, Hjalmarsson & Oertel 2012, Mesch 2016, Oertel et al. 2012, Saubesty & Tellier 2016, Szatrowski 2000) and filled pauses (Beattie 1979, Brône et al. 2017, Kosmala & Morgenstern 2017) and that there is a complex interplay between these modalities in fully natural conversation. Despite these constraints, I am confident that the elicitation method used here constitutes an improvement over those used in related studies and described above, foremost because it enables us to analyse social *interactions* between *disposition-matched* interlocutors (cf. Dingemanse et al. 2023).

Second, the current analysis is limited to a quantitative account, as no analysis of the conversational context of backchannel and filled pause productions can be provided in the scope of this work. Similarly, analysing the interaction of different functional types of hesitations and feedback signals (e.g. passive recipiency vs. incipient speakership) with lexical and prosodic realisation holds promise for future investigations (Jefferson 1984, Jurafsky et al. 1998, Savino 2010, Sbranna et al. 2022, 2023).

Third, a specific methodological limitation concerns the prosodic analysis of BCs and filled pauses. In this account, the difference in pitch between two fixed time points was calculated (near the beginning and the end of each token) to represent intonation contours (having discarded all tokens for which the calculation of pitch was unreliable). As backchannels and filled pauses are very short (<500 ms in almost all cases), this somewhat simplified view does still capture the essential qualities of intonation contours and is perceptually valid. Nevertheless, the method used cannot reliably account for very fine-grained details of intonational realisation and adequately capture more complex contours such as rise–fall–rises. Future investigations might avoid these shortcomings by using more temporally fine-grained techniques such as polynomial modelling (Belz & Reichel 2015), generalised additive mixed modelling (Sóskuthy 2021) or analyses in the ProPer framework (Albert et al. 2018, Albert 2023, Albert et al. 2020, Cangemi et al. 2019). Explorations of the data set under study with the latter two methodologies suggest, however, that the very short durations of individual tokens can be problematic for analysis in at least these frameworks, and that achieving an improvement over the current intonational analysis is therefore not guaranteed. Alternatives to the analysis and modelling of intonation contours will be explored in more detail in forthcoming work.

Finally, a limited sample of subjects from one extreme end of the autism spectrum (verbal, socially relatively skilled and motivated individuals with average or above-average IQ) was investigated for the current work. The data at hand do not allow us to generalise the present findings to interactions between disposition-mixed dyads (ASD–CTR) or to fully spontaneous, multi-modal interaction (see §6.2.6).

6 Conclusion

6.1 Summary analysis

I will start this final part of the book by providing an overview of some key results in the form of a summary analysis, focussing on different dimensions of conversation and intonation in ASD and identifying patterns of dyad-specific behaviour.

This will be followed by a broader discussion of the overarching conclusions we can draw from the large number of results presented in the preceding chapters. Finally, I will attempt to provide a compact synthesis of the most important findings and finish with a brief outlook to future avenues of investigation.

Figure 6.1 presents an overview of results from the key dimensions described in this book for all seven ASD dyads. The primary purpose of this overview table is not to give a comprehensive account of all the results described in preceding chapters, but rather to provide a concise and accessible illustration of the patterns that characterise the behaviour of autistic dyads in the current data set as compared to the CTR group.

	Intonation Style		Turns	Backchannels		Filled Pauses		Silent P.
	Wig.	Spac.	Timing	Rate	Diversity	Rate	Prosody	Rate
F02_F03				+	-		+	
M07_M08	+	+		-	-	+	-	+
M11_F05	+	+						
M04_M05	+	+			-		-	
M06_F04	+		+	-			-	+
M09A_M10A				-	-			
M02_M03				-		+		

Figure 6.1: Overview table for each ASD dyad along five dimensions and eight parameters, as compared to averages from the CTR group. Black cells represent strong effects, grey cells represent moderate effects. See text for further details.

6.1.1 Rationale and parameters

One or two parameters were selected to represent each of the five main dimensions of dialogue management and intonation discussed in the preceding chapters. These parameters were chosen for being at once appropriately representative of the larger phenomenon at hand and conveniently representable in a summary table.

For instance, while for both backchannels and filled pauses, a column for rate of production is included (fourth and sixth column in Figure 6.1), a different second parameter was chosen for each dimension. Prosodic realisation is shown for filled pauses (seventh column), whereas diversity of BC types is shown for backchannels (fifth column). This was done for two complementary reasons. As the difference between the two filled pause types *uh* and *uhm* in prosodic realisation was not robust in the group comparison, it is appropriate to calculate results across types and represent them in a single column. For the same reason, choice of filled pause type is not a particularly informative parameter and is not included in the summary table in Figure 6.1. The reverse is the case for backchannels. As prosodic realisation is specific to each of the four main types of backchannel (*genau* ('exactly'), *ja* ('yeah/yes'), *mmhm* and *okay*), it would be uninformative at best and misleading at worst to present results of prosodic realisation across types in a single column (while the alternative of using four separate columns would defeat the purpose of a summary analysis). Conversely, choice of backchannel type is a highly informative parameter and is therefore represented with a dedicated column showing the diversity of backchannel types produced.

For intonation style, both relevant parameters (Wiggliness and Spaciousness) used in the two-dimensional analysis presented in Chapter 3 are shown (first and second column). For turn-taking, only the single parameter of FTO (Floor Transfer Offset; third column), used as a measure of turn-timing, is shown. FTO suffices to represent all the relevant patterns found in the analysis of turn-taking (presented in Chapter 4). Backchannelling is represented by the parameters of rate and diversity, while production of filled pauses is represented by the parameters of rate and prosodic realisation (as presented in Chapter 5; see above for rationale). Finally, the rate of silent pauses ≥700 milliseconds (as reported in §5.5) is shown in the summary table (eighth column). This parameter complements the analyses of both turn-timing and filled pauses.

Behaviour was analysed at the level of dyads and not speakers, for all parameters. While speaker-specific analyses were used for suitable measures in the preceding chapters, this is not appropriate or even possible for all parameters presented in Figure 6.1. For instance, the rate of backchannels produced by one speaker crucially depends on how many appropriate opportunities for backchannelling the speech of the interlocutor provides, while turn-timing can only be measured in the transitional space between talk by two interlocutors.

Cells in the summary table are filled in and colour-coded to represent divergence from (average) behaviour in the CTR group. Strong effects are defined as any mean values by (ASD) dyad that fell outside the range of the mean of the CTR group ±1 standard deviation (i.e. outside the central 68% of values). Such effects are represented with black cells, with "+" or "-" icons representing the direction of the effect.

Moderate effects (grey cells) are defined as any mean values by dyad that were higher (+) or lower (-) than the average of any single CTR dyad. If a mean value fulfilled the criteria for both strong and moderate effects (as was occasionally the case), the effect is considered to be strong. Details of the resulting cut-off values for each parameter along with summary tables can be found in the accompanying *OSF* repository (https://osf.io/6vynj/).

I have avoided relying on inferential statistical tests to characterise divergences in the behaviour of the ASD dyads in this summary analysis, in keeping with the emphasis on thorough, transparent description that I have followed throughout this book (see §2.3). It was confirmed that the heuristic thresholds chosen are representative of the results from Bayesian modelling and of the in-depth dyad- and speaker-specific analyses previously performed for all parameters and dimensions.

6.1.2 Identification and interpretation of dyad-specific patterns

Overall, we can observe that no column and no row in the summary table is either completely filled or completely empty and, moreover, that no two columns or rows are identical to each other. In other words, all ASD dyads diverged from average behaviour in the CTR group in their own unique way and along different parameters. While all dyads clearly diverged from CTR behaviour in some regards, none did so along all parameters.

This is simply another way of highlighting the fundamental fact that dyad-specific (or individual-specific) behaviour is a crucial aspect of spoken communication, and that we ignore this fact in favour of simplified group-level analyses at the peril of scientific integrity and descriptive accuracy. Studying a group of individuals with ASD is a particularly suitable test case for this assertion (due to the characteristically high inter-individual variability), but the principle holds for studies of non-autistic speakers (cf. §2.3.1 and §6.2.1).

Considering the different dimensions of analysis (columns in Figure 6.1), we can see that the CTR and ASD groups differed most clearly in their use of backchannels (with strong effects for six out of seven dyads). The greatest similarity between groups, on the other hand, can be found in turn-timing behaviour (with only one dyad showing a (moderate) effect). The remaining dimensions fall in between these two poles, with at least moderate differences in intonation style for most dyads, mixed results for filled pauses (more differences for prosodic realisation than rate) and a (strong) difference in silent pause rate for two out of seven dyads.

As we shift our attention to dyad-specific behaviour (rows in Figure 6.1), the most immediate observation is that there is a "lack of invariance" within the ASD group, to borrow a term from speech perception (Liberman et al. 1967). In other words, we find further evidence for a great degree of heterogeneity across the behaviour of different individuals (and dyads) diagnosed with ASD. In the following paragraphs, I will briefly describe the patterns observed for each ASD dyad. The relevant overview plots can be found in the folder "turnation" of the accompanying *OSF* repository at https://osf.io/6vynj/.

Dyad F02_F03 (top row) produced notable differences from average CTR behaviour for two out of five dimensions and three out of eight parameters. This pair of speakers did not notably differ from the CTR average in terms of intonation style, turn-taking and silent pause rate. Regarding filled pauses, there was a moderate effect for prosodic realisation (more rising tokens, with the highest mean value out of all dyads – all other ASD dyads produced lower or equivalent values), but not for rate.

The clearest differences were found for the dimension of backchannelling. F02_F03 was the only ASD dyad to produce a *higher* rate of backchannels (the second highest overall) than the CTR average (with a strong effect). Out of the remaining six ASD dyads, four dyads had a lower rate and two dyads had a rate comparable to the CTR average. Besides the lower rate, F02_F03 also produced a reduced variety of different backchannel types (strong effect).

This pattern of behaviour is highly salient perceptually, as it results in dialogue containing a very high number of very similar backchannels, e.g. "*ja....ja....ja*". Not shown in the summary table is the fact that, additionally, these productions were also not very diverse in terms of prosodic realisation, as almost all tokens (across types) in this dyad were produced with rising intonation (cf. Figure 5.11). Backchannels also seemed to be produced at quite regular intervals and independent of conversational context. This last aspect remains an impressionistic observation at this point, as the exact timing of backchannels was not analysed. The overview plot (in the repository) gives an idea of the frequency and timing of backchannel tokens (particularly noticeable in the form of the light blue dots in the second half of dialogue).

The overview plot also illustrates that the speakers in dyad F02_F03 seemed to adhere rather closely to their assigned roles of instruction follower and giver, as each half of the dialogue consists mostly of speech by the instruction giver. Instruction followers responded mostly with very short utterances (i.e. backchannels in most cases), especially in the second half of the task. This conversational style is further reflected in the facts that 1) overall dialogue duration was very short (the second shortest overall) and 2) this dyad was the only one to essentially ignore the fact that there were mismatching landmarks between the two participants' maps (the issue was noted, but not discussed before the participants immediately moved on to a description of the next part of the map; see green outline in the overview plot).

Dyad M07_M08 (second row) was the dyad to diverge most clearly overall from the CTR average, showing notable differences along all five dimensions and for seven out of eight parameters. The only dimension for which no notable difference was detected is turn-timing. Intonation style in this dyad was more melodic than in the CTR average, with moderate effects of both higher Wiggliness (the highest value of all dyads) and Spaciousness (the third highest value overall). Strong effects were also found for backchannelling, with a low diversity of BC types as well as a low rate of BCs produced (the lowest out of all dyads; see leftmost square in Figure 5.1). Finally, strong effects were found in a higher rate of silent pauses (the highest rate overall) and filled pauses (the third highest rate overall), as well as a moderate effect in the prosodic realisation of filled pauses (more falling; with the lowest mean value out of all dyads).

Impressionistically, these divergences along different dimensions have a cumulative effect, leading to a notably unusual conversation style. For instance, a short exchange between M07 and M08 might not only contain few backchannels or none at all, but at the same time feature many silent *and* filled pauses (the latter somewhat unusual in prosodic form as well). Additionally, task duration was rather short and speaking times were not well-balanced between interlocutors (with a score of 17%; cf. §4.4.4.3). There are no obvious a priori reasons for the extent of divergence in this particular dyad. Both speakers were well within the range of individuals within the ASD group as regards age, AQ and verbal IQ.

Dyad M11_F05 (third row) stands in direct contrast to dyad M07_M08 (discussed directly above), as this pair of speakers produced the least amount of notable differences from the CTR average out of all ASD dyads. Behaviour was comparable to typical patterns in the CTR group for all dimensions except for both parameters characterising intonation style (moderate effects of both higher

Wiggliness and higher Spaciousness). Just as for M07_M08, there are no obvious a priori reasons to suggest why this dyad might stand out from the other dyads within the ASD group. It is interesting to note, however, that dialogue in this speaker pair actually started off in a very unusual fashion, with only minimal verbal contributions by the instruction follower in the first couple of minutes. This changed after an explicit statement by the instruction giver encouraging the interlocutor to comment on his instructions and to ask questions (around minute 2:45).

Dyad M04_M05 (fourth row) produced notable differences from average CTR behaviour along three out of five dimensions and four out of eight parameters. These differences mostly concerned prosodic aspects. M04_M05 was the only speaker pair to show a strong effect for differences in intonation style, with the highest overall Spaciousness value. There was also a moderate effect for higher Wiggliness, representing the second highest value out of all dyads.

M04_M05 produced the second lowest value for prosodic realisation of filled pauses (i.e. more falling contours; moderate effect) and the lowest diversity of backchannels (strong effect). All these differences are perceptually particularly salient because task duration was the shortest out of all recorded dyads (under 9 minutes). No differences in turn-timing were found, nor for the rates of backchannels, filled pauses and silent pauses.

Dyad M06_F04 (fifth row) is the second dyad (along with M07_M08) to show notable differences for all five dimensions (five out of eight parameters). This dyad stands out in particular as being the only dyad with a clear difference in turn-timing compared to average CTR behaviour, with the highest mean value of all dyads (moderate effect). The speaker pair showed moderate effects for Wiggliness (higher than CTR average) and the prosodic realisation of filled pauses (lower than CTR average). Further, strong effects were found in a higher rate of silent pauses and a lower rate of backchannels.

The cumulative effect of longer between-speaker gaps, more frequent long within-speaker pauses and fewer backchannels is perceptually quite salient and manifests as an unusual overall proportion of silence in the dialogue, visible as a comparatively large amount of white space in the overview plot (in the repository). The overview plot also illustrates a pattern of interlocutors adhering rather strictly to their assigned roles of instruction follower and instruction giver in each Map Task.

Dyad M09A_M10A (sixth row) was one of two dyads (along with M11_F05) to differ from average CTR behaviour for only one single dimension (and two parameters), in this case, backchannelling. M09A_M10A produced the second lowest rate and diversity of backchannel tokens (both strong effects). Behaviour was comparable to the CTR average for all other parameters. This dyad was notable also for having the longest dialogue duration out of all ASD dyads by a large margin (30 minutes – 13 minutes more than the next longest dialogue, by ASD dyad M11_F05).

Thereby, the two ASD dyads with the longest dialogue durations were also the two that only showed divergence from average CTR behaviour along one single dimension. We can only speculate about the significance (if any) of this correlation, but it is tempting to connect this to the suggestion that the combination of shorter overall dialogues in the ASD group combined with proportionately fewer backchannels and less laughter might indicate a more goal-oriented and efficient (at least from a functional perspective) conversation style (see the discussion of backchannels in §5.7.1). Conversely, longer dialogues such as by dyads M09A_-M10A and M11_F05 might be indicative of a more explicitly other-oriented and affiliative conversation style.

Finally, dyad M02_M03 (bottom row) showed relatively few divergences from average CTR behaviour. Specifically, the differences identified were a lower rate of backchannels and the highest filled pause rate of all dyads (both strong effects). Once again, these are clearly not orthogonal effects, but rather, their interaction can be expected to have a cumulative effect on the holistic perception of conversational style. Backchannels and filled pauses have directly contrasting functions (as discussed in §5.4.1 and §5.7.3). Backchannels are used by listeners to support the turn of the other speaker, while filled pauses are used by speakers to prolong their own turn and avoid transferring the floor. Thus the higher rate of filled pauses and lower rate of backchannels in dyad M02_M03 add up to the (impressionistic) sense that both speakers were focussed much more on their own turns at talk than they were on encouraging their interlocutor to speak.

Fittingly, this pair of speakers adhered to the roles of instruction giver and follower comparatively strictly (see overview plot in the repository), possibly reflecting a prioritisation of orderly completion of the task over spontaneous engagement with the interlocutor (see description of dyad M09A_M10A above for discussion and further examples).

6.1.3 Limitations of the summary analysis

I already mentioned in the introduction that this summary analysis is not intended to be, and indeed cannot be, an exhaustive overview of all the communicative behaviours examined in this book. Rather, it represents my best attempt to reduce the considerable amount of complexity that is common to the manifold aspects of conversation and intonation covered in this work to an easily digestible whole.

Although a certain degree of simplification was necessary to achieve this aim, I believe that this overview still accurately represents the essence of the key findings presented in this work. I have been as transparent as possible about the fact that a number of subjective decisions were made regarding the inclusion and exclusion of various parameters as well as the setting of thresholds for what are considered moderate or strong effects. Although I have made every effort to ascertain that the specific choices made were best suited to this compact yet representative analysis, it should be self-evident that such choices are always debatable and can have a considerable impact on the outcome of any analysis (Coretta et al. 2023, Roettger 2019).

One corollary of concentrating the summary analysis on an easy-to-process number of dimensions was that results were considered across the entire duration of dialogues. It is thereby not possible to acknowledge some of the intriguing patterns that were found by comparing early with later stages of dialogue here. The reader is referred to the relevant sections in the preceding chapters (e.g. §4.4.1.3 and §5.3.2.1) as well as in the concluding remarks (§6.2.4) for more details on the comparison of different dialogue stages.

One further general and potentially problematic limitation of this summary analysis is the fact that, for this specific purpose only, the CTR group was considered as a monolithic whole. This was done in order to identify group means which would serve as reference values in the comparison with ASD dyads. As discussed at length in the immediately preceding section, however, the most important message from this summary analysis concerns the supreme importance of appropriately considering and accounting for inter-individual and dyad-specific variability in the study of human behaviour. While this assertion might seem to stand in direct opposition to the method of quantifying ASD–CTR differences in this summary analysis, I submit that it is more fruitful to formulate a certain number of carefully considered generalisations *along with* detailed, dyad/speaker-specific analyses than to avoid doing so as a matter of principle. In this light, the reader is explicitly encouraged to not only critically question the choices made in this work, but to also independently follow alternative paths of analysis using the data and code provided in the accompanying files.

6.2 General discussion

I would like to conclude with a brief summary of the most important findings and by adding some final thoughts on possible implications as well as interpretation and contextualisation.

6.2.1 Autistic persons as particularly individual individuals

Throughout this book, I have acknowledged the importance of individual specificity to not only my own field of study, but also related ones. I determined from the outset to focus on individual- and dyad-specific behaviour in sufficient detail to arrive at an accurate description at the group level, all the more so in the case of the ASD group. The analytical choice of emphasising transparent, in-depth description at the levels of individuals, dyads and groups supported by Bayesian modelling reflects this stance.

I emphasised throughout that overlap between the ASD and the CTR group was found for each single one out of the dozens of parameters investigated in this multi-dimensional analysis of conversation and intonation. It was further shown that group means usually do not suffice to accurately portray the underlying behaviour of the individuals and dyads within a group. Finally, considerable evidence has been amassed to further strengthen the well-established argument that individual differences play a particularly important role in ASD (cf. Grice et al. 2023, Goldberg & Abbot-Smith 2021, Wozniak et al. 2017). Even in the slightly simplified summary analysis presented in §6.1, there is not a single dimension or parameter for which the behaviour of all seven autistic dyads was the same or equivalent.

Having performed in-depth analysis at the level of individuals and dyads ultimately also enables us to more confidently formulate generalisations at the group-level. These generalisations never apply equally to each autistic dyad in the current sample (or beyond), but they do give us some strong hints about robust tendencies of behaviour. This is all the more valuable in the description of a group as broad and varied as that of individuals diagnosed with ASD. I will discuss some of the most important general observations and conclusions in the following sections.

6.2.2 Backchannelling as a prototype of other-oriented communicative behaviour

The clearest overall difference between groups was found for backchannelling. Six out of seven autistic dyads clearly diverged from typical behaviour in the control group for this dimension. As mentioned previously, backchannels are distinguished by being a relatively implicit and decidedly pro-social communicative signal. The specific finding of, for instance, a reduced rate of backchannels might reflect a more general lack of interest in explicitly showing attention to an interlocutor by autistic individuals (but keep in mind that the group difference was very clear only for the earliest stages of dialogue; see §6.2.4 below). The simple to calculate metric of backchannels per minute might thus serve as a reliable correlate of general tendencies in autistic communication.

A reduced rate of backchannels in ASD can be related to what has been described in previous studies for the behaviour of non-autistic speakers in task-oriented as opposed to free conversation. As pointed out in other parts of this book, a lower rate of backchannels, especially when combined with related findings, e.g. the fact that dialogues in the ASD group were shorter and contained less laughter, seems to point to an approach to social interaction that prioritises efficiency. In other words, the analyses reported in this book seem to reveal specific behavioural correlates of an autistic preference for goal-oriented communication. It is interesting to note that backchannels have historically often been described as a non-essential and functionally irrelevant element of language – largely owing to an overemphasis on written language and/or monologic speech in the dominant theoretical and pedagogical approaches (Linell 2004, Schegloff 1982, O'Connell & Kowal 2004). It might be no coincidence that backchannels seem to play a diminished role in the perception and communicative style of a group that often priorities explicitness and economy over small talk and purely affiliative aspects of social interaction.

Measuring the diversity of backchannel types is a little less straightforward than measuring their rate, but the relevant finding of reduced diversity in the ASD group can be promisingly linked to the other main diagnostic criterion for ASD besides difficulties in social communication, i.e. circumscribed or inflexible behaviour.

The fact that backchannel behaviour in ASD has not been investigated in any detail to date makes it highly promising overall as an additional component in the description and assessment of autistic communication styles in future.

6.2.3 Turn-timing as a fundamental and universal skill in interaction

In direct contrast to backchannelling, hardly any consistent overall differences were found regarding the turn-timing of autistic as compared to non-autistic dyads. Only one out of seven ASD dyads showed a notable difference in global turn-timing, and even this difference was rather slight. While I have described backchannels as implicit and affiliative signals, a rapid exchange of turns is evidently essential for any functioning coordinated interaction with the speed and complexity of spoken dialogue. Turn-taking is a fundamental aspect of social interaction and the relevant skills are not limited to the use of language. In this sense it is not entirely surprising that the current findings serve to add speakers on the autism spectrum to the many diverse groups of speakers who, despite manifold cognitive, cultural and linguistic differences, have been found to exhibit remarkably similar turn-timing behaviour.

While the experimental task of transferring a route from the map of one person to that of another without visual contact could in principle be accomplished without the production of any backchannels, it would be all but impossible to do so without the rapid exchange of spoken utterances. Additionally, any lengthy transitions containing overlapping speech or between-speaker silence are not only likely to be perceived as awkward or unusual, but would also reduce the efficiency of the communicative exchange at a purely functional level. Thus, fast and effective turn-timing does not require a decidedly social motivation in the same way that frequent backchannelling does.

6.2.4 Initial differences as a reflection of effortful accommodation

Social motivations aside, achieving the speed of turn-timing found in typical conversations between adult native speakers remains a formidable challenge and requires complex social skills, such as the accurate prediction of an interlocutor's behaviour. Predicting others becomes easier the more familiar interlocutors are with each other and the more two (or more) speakers establish a shared conversational rhythm in the sense of convergence or accommodation. I have speculatively interpreted the observation that ASD dyads take considerably longer to achieve typically rapid turn-timing as signifying a delay in the establishment of a shared rhythm and a concordantly high degree of convergence between interlocutors.

A similar effect was observed for backchannelling. The rate of backchannels goes up rather steeply for most ASD dyads as conversations progress and thereby becomes much more similar to the values typically produced by CTR dyads. Thus, dyads from the ASD group often arrived at behaviour comparable to that of the CTR group after the first few minutes of conversation, suggesting that it was only a matter of time for autistic dyads to reach the level of coordination that is typical for conversation in the CTR group. This delay could be an indication that superficially equivalent behaviour between groups at a global level may obscure the fact that arriving at these behaviours may be more effortful for some autistic individuals. In this light, one reason why conversations in the ASD group were comparatively short and to the point – besides any potential lack of social motivation – would simply be increased cognitive effort.

Taking different stages of conversation into account has thus yielded some valuable insights that would otherwise have been overlooked. Paying special attention to the early stages of dialogue is particularly important since previous research has reliably shown that personality judgements and character attributions are disproportionately influenced by the first minutes and even seconds of a social interaction. This implies that although the behaviour of autistic dyads might be equivalent to that of non-autistic dyads for the majority of a conversation, diverging behaviour in the early stages of conversation may nevertheless leave indelible impressions of an unconventional communication style.

6.2.5 Intonation as a global and local feature of speech

Differences between early and later stages of dialogue were not found for all areas of investigation. Intonation styles in particular are noteworthy for having remained stable throughout the task for almost all speakers. This suggests that intonation styles are a global property of speakers and largely robust to external factors such as context and content. It is therefore particularly relevant that a clear indication for only more melodic (or singsongy), but not more monotonous (or robotic) intonation in ASD dyads was found, adding to the mounting evidence that a melodic intonation style is characteristic of speech in ASD.

Prosodic aspects of speech and differences between groups were investigated not only at the global level of intonation styles, but also as part of the local realisation of backchannels and filled pauses (as well as turn ends and beginnings). For backchannels, it was found that the mapping of intonation contours to different lexical types of backchannel was less complex in the ASD group than in the CTR group. In essence, many ASD dyads showed a preference for rising intonation contours on all lexical types of BC, whereas most CTR dyads evinced a more specific probabilistic mapping of intonation contour to BC type. For filled pauses (the rate of which was identical across groups), realisations by ASD dyads deviated more from the expected level contour than those by CTR dyads.

Accurately employing prosody in the production of backchannels and filled pauses requires an acute understanding of the rather subtle ways in which not only one class of discourse marker (BC) differs from the other (FP), but also of the commonly preferred contours for different types *within* the class of backchannels. The reduced degree of complexity shown by most ASD dyads in the prosodic realisation of BCs might conceivably be linked to the typically less restrained use of intonation at the global level, manifesting as a more melodic intonation style.

6.2.6 The autistic sample as a filter on the spectrum

It is important to remember that all the differences between groups that have been described and all the characteristics of conversation in ASD that have been inferred from these differences are based on a very specific and limited sample. Not only were the participants in the ASD group German-speaking, mostly male and considerably older than the average experimental subject in linguistics and psychology. Most importantly, they were far from representative of the autism spectrum as a whole. Through a largely implicit selection procedure, participants were required to be 1) verbal, 2) willing and able to visit an outpatient clinic, 3) of average or above-average intelligence and 4) willing and able to take part in an unfamiliar experiment (in an unfamiliar location and wearing head-mounted microphones). These requirements act as a narrow-band filter, leaving us with behavioural data from only one peripheral region within the entire autism spectrum.

As this places the experimental subjects in the ASD group very close to the point where individuals with and without a diagnosis of ASD (the latter represented by the CTR group in the corpus under investigation) are most likely to overlap, it is perhaps all the more remarkable that such varied differences between groups were found. Had the CTR group consisted of subjects from the stereotypical linguistics subject pool of female undergraduate students, even more or clearer differences between groups may well have been found, but it would not have been possible to attribute them specifically to a difference in autistic traits. Given that the CTR group was instead carefully matched for gender, age and verbal IQ, the patterns of behaviour that were identified as typical for the ASD group are likely to indeed be specific to an autistic communication style. We have to keep in mind, however, that the small sample size of 14 subjects, while relatively high compared to other studies on autistic communication, necessarily limits external validity.

Studying individuals from one narrow band along the autism spectrum crucially also entails not being able to make predictions about individuals from the rest of the spectrum. It is worth stating explicitly that the findings in this work cannot be expected to generalise to the majority of autistic people, many of whom might have been unwilling or unable to take part in the recordings and complete the experimental task. Even though terms such as "high-functioning autism" or even "Asperger syndrome" have, with some justification, fallen out of favour and indeed use in recent years (see §1.1), the findings described in this book may most accurately represent the behaviour of adults matching just those descriptions. It bears repeating that I cannot and do not wish to make any claims regarding children and/or individuals on other parts of the autism spectrum on the basis of the work presented here, nor do I claim that the methodology used would be suitable for the study of communication in these groups.

6.2.7 Bilingual and cross-cultural conversation as a valuable analogy

Partly due to a lack of previous research into autistic communication, I have used results from research on second language learners and bilinguals to contextualise results from the group of autistic subjects under study in various parts of this book. I have tried to make it sufficiently clear that there are crucial differences between autistic and non-native speakers and that I focus on similarities between the two groups as an approximate analogy only (see e.g. §1.1). I do believe, however, that much could be gained in theory and practice from connecting the two fields of study.

Communication between autistic and non-autistic individuals could reasonably be seen as an analogue of cross-cultural communication. Interestingly, individuals with ASD often feel more at ease in cross-cultural social contexts, as in such situations, communicative difficulties are usually expected and tend not to be ascribed to a failing on the part of only one interlocutor (Hillary 2020). This relates directly to the concept of the double empathy problem (discussed in several parts of the book), i.e. essentially the idea that difficulties in communication between autistic and non-autistic speakers are mainly due to divergent social dispositions. This again entails that difficulties in communication are created in the interaction between two interlocutors, an idea closely related to that of a shared responsibility between native and non-native speakers proposed in e.g. Derwing & Munro (2009). Following this line of thought, there is a strong case to be made for putting the onus on non-autistic individuals to make every effort to understand and accommodate autistic styles of communication and cognition (cf. McCracken 2021).

To be able to do so, we of course first need to gain a much more accurate idea of what can be considered as truly autistic styles of conversation and intonation, which will require many more studies of disposition-matched autistic communication to be conducted in future. The present book represents my contribution to this effort. Specific results described here could also be used to fine-tune the analogy of autistic with non-native or bilingual speech. For instance, the current findings on intonation style, turn-taking and backchannelling much more closely resemble previous findings on bilinguals or *near-native* learners (Sorace 2003) than findings on beginner learners, as might be expected given the specific sample of the autistic population, that is, individuals from the more socially motivated and skilled end of the spectrum.

Finally, I will point out the great potential for adapting research, teaching and training materials from second-language instruction and inter-cultural training to the study of communication between autistic and non-autistic people. The more we are able to pinpoint what characterises communication in ASD, the more we will be able to tap into the vast array of relevant resources and adapt them for the benefit of anyone who is engaged or merely interested in understanding and facilitating communication between autistic and non-autistic individuals.

6.3 Outlook

I will close by summarising some of the most important projected extensions of the work described in this book.

First, follow-up production studies which are already under way include video recordings, making it possible to examine the contributions of gesture and gaze to conversational strategies and their interplay with the spoken modality (see the pilot study in Spaniol et al. 2023).

Second, experimental settings have been extended to include fully free (but also highly structured) conversations (Spaniol et al. 2023).

Third, mixed dyads (ASD–CTR) should be included to compare the relevant interactions with what has been described here for disposition-matched (ASD–ASD/CTR–CTR) dyads. This could involve the analysis of triadic rather than dyadic interaction, which incidentally facilitates tracking the contributions of individual speakers to social interaction. A comparison with conversation and intonation in persons with schizophrenia furthermore holds promise for future investigations (cf. Lucarini et al. 2021, Cangemi et al. 2023, Howes et al. 2017). A comparison of autistic individuals from different age ranges or ideally even longitudinal observations throughout development would be highly valuable, if logistically challenging extensions.

Fourth, improvements can be made on specific methods of analysis used, e.g. by including periodic energy or polynomial modelling in the analysis of prosody and by considering convergence continuously across the time course of conversations.

Fifth, perception studies can help us to critically examine and further refine the measures and findings described in this work. For instance, experiments can verify how closely the analysis of intonation styles proposed in this work matches listener impressions (see a first validation in Wehrle & Sappok 2023) and shed light on how conversational strategies specific to the ASD group are perceived and judged by both autistic and non-autistic listeners.

Finally, qualitative analyses and insights from autistic adults will be used to shape the interpretation of current and future results. The insights and experiences shared by the participants of the FORAUS discussion forum for autistic adults in Cologne, for instance, have been invaluable for understanding and contextualising the quantitative analyses reported throughout this book. I will continue the exchange with autistic informants and advocates to ensure that the lived experiences of autistic people are represented appropriately, and to inform future efforts of raising broader societal awareness of communication in ASD.

Once the findings presented in this book have been subject to further critical examination and, ideally, replication efforts in future studies, we will be better able to assess their relevance and suitability for applications in, for instance, training and diagnosis. For the time being, it is my hope that this work has added to our general understanding of conversation and intonation in ASD by shedding light on some of the most important underlying dimensions and mechanisms. Ultimately, I hope that the findings presented in this work might help to contribute to an acceptance of neurodiversity in highlighting ASD-specific communication strategies and their potential relevance for cross-neurotype communication.

Appendix A: Intonation style

Table A.1 shows results for intonation styles by speaker, gender and group (ordered by dyad). Tables A.2 and A.3 show results for mean f0 by gender and group (A.2) as well as individual speakers (A.3; ordered by dyad). Table A.4 shows results for intonation styles by part of dialogue (in chronological order) and by dyad. Note that for three speakers, values are not reported for all parts of the dialogue. In these cases, no suitable speech data were available due to the fact that no utterances with a duration of at least 1 second were produced in the relevant part of the task. Figure A.1 shows results for intonation style by speaker and role (instruction giver vs. instruction follower).

Table A.1: Intonation style by speaker. Spaciousness in semitones; SD = standard deviation.

			Wiggliness		Spaciousness	
Group	Speaker	Gender	Mean	SD	Mean	SD
ASD	F02	Female	3.31	1.13	5.58	2.25
ASD	F03	Female	3.13	0.91	5.58	2.25
ASD	F05	Female	3.79	0.92	8.64	2.14
ASD	M11	Male	3.42	0.96	7.52	2.11
ASD	M07	Male	3.77	1.03	7.24	2.42
ASD	M08	Male	4.11	1.11	6.48	1.90
ASD	M04	Male	3.69	1.09	9.21	2.27
ASD	M05	Male	3.90	1.12	8.48	2.78
ASD	M06	Male	3.63	1.12	5.99	2.24
ASD	F04	Female	3.38	0.90	7.47	2.35
ASD	M09A	Male	2.76	0.98	5.70	2.24
ASD	M10A	Male	3.37	0.89	5.98	1.77
ASD	M02	Male	3.15	0.96	5.78	2.52
ASD	M03	Male	3.03	1.06	5.79	2.19
CTR	F20	Female	2.78	0.98	5.23	2.12
CTR	M13	Male	3.44	1.19	7.32	2.66
CTR	F21	Female	3.38	0.99	6.57	2.00
CTR	M14	Male	3.63	1.01	7.11	2.29
CTR	F23	Female	2.64	0.82	4.92	1.96
CTR	M22	Male	2.93	1.10	4.78	1.98
CTR	M09	Male	2.92	1.02	6.33	2.55
CTR	M10	Male	3.27	1.01	6.79	2.42
CTR	M11C	Male	3.11	1.10	5.91	2.24
CTR	M12	Male	2.54	0.82	5.38	1.89
CTR	M15	Male	2.53	0.90	4.61	1.99
CTR	M16	Male	3.30	1.07	5.55	2.05
CTR	M18	Male	2.99	0.97	5.57	2.26
CTR	M19	Male	3.05	1.03	4.85	2.03

Table A.2: Mean f0 values by gender and group (in Hz).

Gender	Group	Mean f0	SD
Female	ASD	224.50	8.32
Female	CTR	233.70	8.85
Male	ASD	136.03	17.55
Male	CTR	126.50	18.26

Table A.3: Mean f0 values by speaker (in Hz; ordered by dyad).

Group	Speaker	Gender	Mean f0	SD
ASD	F02	Female	218.27	35.24
ASD	F03	Female	232.44	33.70
ASD	F05	Female	230.86	44.84
ASD	M11	Male	148.34	36.56
ASD	M07	Male	135.70	31.39
ASD	M08	Male	171.61	30.65
ASD	M04	Male	149.57	35.13
ASD	M05	Male	110.45	27.17
ASD	M06	Male	133.52	25.13
ASD	F04	Female	216.42	50.98
ASD	M09A	Male	138.20	26.65
ASD	M10A	Male	131.86	24.93
ASD	M02	Male	122.27	25.06
ASD	M03	Male	118.74	20.50
CTR	F20	Female	243.74	40.34
CTR	M13	Male	121.46	30.62
CTR	F21	Female	227.02	45.36
CTR	M14	Male	156.09	33.73
CTR	F23	Female	230.33	41.09
CTR	M22	Male	118.43	19.93
CTR	M09	Male	156.37	33.37
CTR	M10	Male	126.76	28.79
CTR	M11C	Male	114.32	21.05
CTR	M12	Male	107.76	18.09
CTR	M15	Male	133.70	24.46
CTR	M16	Male	136.13	27.14
CTR	M18	Male	122.56	24.08
CTR	M19	Male	97.95	16.05

Table A.4: Intonation style by part of dialogue and dyad.

			Wiggliness		Spaciousness	
Group	Speaker	Mismatch 1	Mean	SD	Mean	SD
ASD	F02	before	3.38	0.97	6.04	1.39
ASD	F02	during	3.06	NA	5.32	NA
ASD	F02	after	3.30	1.18	5.49	2.40
ASD	F03	after	3.13	0.91	5.58	2.25
ASD	F05	before	3.61	0.52	8.02	1.55
ASD	F05	during	3.99	0.87	8.50	2.19
ASD	F05	after	3.74	0.99	8.80	2.21
ASD	M11	before	2.84	0.73	7.81	2.20
ASD	M11	during	3.24	0.55	7.87	2.07
ASD	M11	after	3.68	0.99	7.34	2.09
ASD	M07	before	3.85	1.13	7.77	2.74
ASD	M07	during	3.48	1.05	7.47	2.42
ASD	M07	after	3.85	0.99	6.99	2.33
ASD	M08	before	4.02	1.04	6.30	1.45
ASD	M08	during	3.96	1.01	6.27	1.77
ASD	M08	after	4.18	1.17	6.60	2.03
ASD	M04	before	5.97	NA	8.67	NA
ASD	M04	during	3.30	1.48	6.86	0.29
ASD	M04	after	3.66	1.03	9.38	2.28
ASD	M05	before	2.89	0.53	12.39	3.13
ASD	M05	during	4.10	1.35	7.24	2.39
ASD	M05	after	3.96	1.04	8.42	2.46
ASD	M06	before	4.09	1.15	6.26	2.19
ASD	M06	during	3.77	1.31	6.12	2.61
ASD	M06	after	3.46	1.06	5.89	2.25
ASD	F04	during	3.12	0.59	8.58	2.89
ASD	F04	after	3.40	0.91	7.40	2.31
ASD	M09A	before	3.24	0.83	6.17	1.61
ASD	M09A	during	2.94	0.95	5.75	2.27
ASD	M09A	after	2.68	0.98	5.67	2.25
ASD	M10A	before	3.31	0.74	5.36	1.04
ASD	M10A	during	3.37	1.08	5.19	1.70
ASD	M10A	after	3.38	0.88	6.13	1.80
ASD	M02	before	3.01	1.08	6.53	3.10

Table A.4 continued

			Wiggliness		Spaciousness	
Group	Speaker	Mismatch 1	Mean	SD	Mean	SD
ASD	M02	during	3.33	0.98	6.81	2.77
ASD	M02	after	3.14	0.91	5.09	1.92
ASD	M03	before	2.56	1.39	3.88	1.21
ASD	M03	during	3.14	1.02	5.15	2.01
ASD	M03	after	3.08	1.01	6.15	2.17
CTR	F20	before	1.87	0.30	3.98	3.01
CTR	F20	during	2.54	0.73	5.00	1.60
CTR	F20	after	2.85	1.01	5.30	2.17
CTR	M13	before	3.42	1.15	7.22	2.20
CTR	M13	during	3.34	1.39	7.09	2.86
CTR	M13	after	3.47	1.15	7.41	2.70
CTR	F21	before	2.94	0.84	6.42	1.88
CTR	F21	during	3.30	0.87	5.92	2.14
CTR	F21	after	3.46	1.04	6.82	1.92
CTR	M14	before	3.66	0.89	7.08	2.59
CTR	M14	during	3.83	1.27	7.35	1.98
CTR	M14	after	3.53	0.94	7.03	2.29
CTR	F23	before	3.04	0.90	5.20	2.00
CTR	F23	during	2.91	0.74	4.06	1.44
CTR	F23	after	2.58	0.81	4.97	1.99
CTR	M22	before	3.20	1.10	4.96	1.67
CTR	M22	during	2.87	0.79	5.18	2.25
CTR	M22	after	2.84	1.15	4.63	2.05
CTR	M09	before	1.95	0.42	4.45	2.63
CTR	M09	during	2.82	0.96	5.98	2.81
CTR	M09	after	2.95	1.03	6.40	2.51
CTR	M10	during	3.50	1.16	7.09	2.66
CTR	M10	after	3.26	1.00	6.77	2.40
CTR	M11C	before	3.45	0.63	6.08	1.83
CTR	M11C	during	3.35	1.27	6.00	1.83
CTR	M11C	after	2.98	1.05	5.85	2.46
CTR	M12	before	2.30	0.52	5.11	2.10
CTR	M12	during	2.69	1.00	5.66	2.01
CTR	M12	after	2.56	0.81	5.34	1.74

Table A.4 continued

			Wiggliness		Spaciousness	
Group	Speaker	Mismatch 1	Mean	SD	Mean	SD
CTR	M15	before	2.82	0.93	5.02	2.11
CTR	M15	during	3.08	0.92	3.97	0.56
CTR	M15	after	2.44	0.87	4.51	1.97
CTR	M16	before	2.80	1.01	4.86	1.81
CTR	M16	during	2.76	0.94	4.62	1.23
CTR	M16	after	3.38	1.07	5.66	2.08
CTR	M18	before	3.01	0.88	6.05	2.56
CTR	M18	during	3.39	1.02	5.81	2.37
CTR	M18	after	2.90	0.95	5.45	2.19
CTR	M19	before	3.30	0.85	5.45	1.97
CTR	M19	during	2.31	0.80	4.13	2.47
CTR	M19	after	3.02	1.08	4.69	1.98

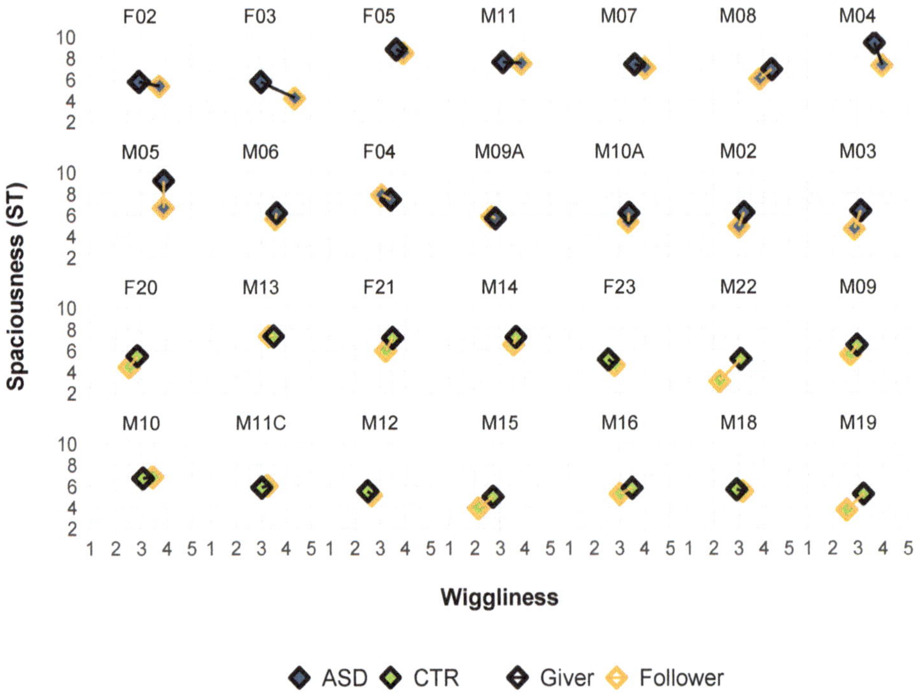

Figure A.1: Intonation style by group and speaker role. Spaciousness on the y-axis (in ST), Wiggliness on the x-axis. ASD speakers in the top two rows, CTR speakers in the bottom two rows (ASD group in blue, CTR group in green). Values for instruction givers are presented with black outlines, values for instruction followers with orange outlines.

Appendix B: Turn-taking

Figure B.1 shows turn-timing values by group in a histogram with 100 ms bins (to match the analysis in Levinson & Torreira 2015). Figure B.2 shows the categorical analysis of transition types by group and dyad. Figure B.3 shows proportions of silence, overlap and single-speaker speech by dyad.

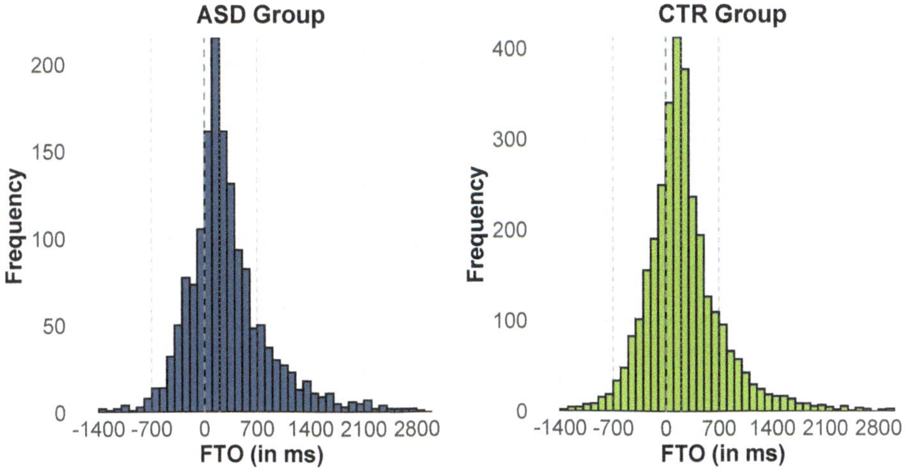

Figure B.1: Histograms of FTO values for the ASD group in the left panel and the CTR group in the right panel (bin width = 100 ms).

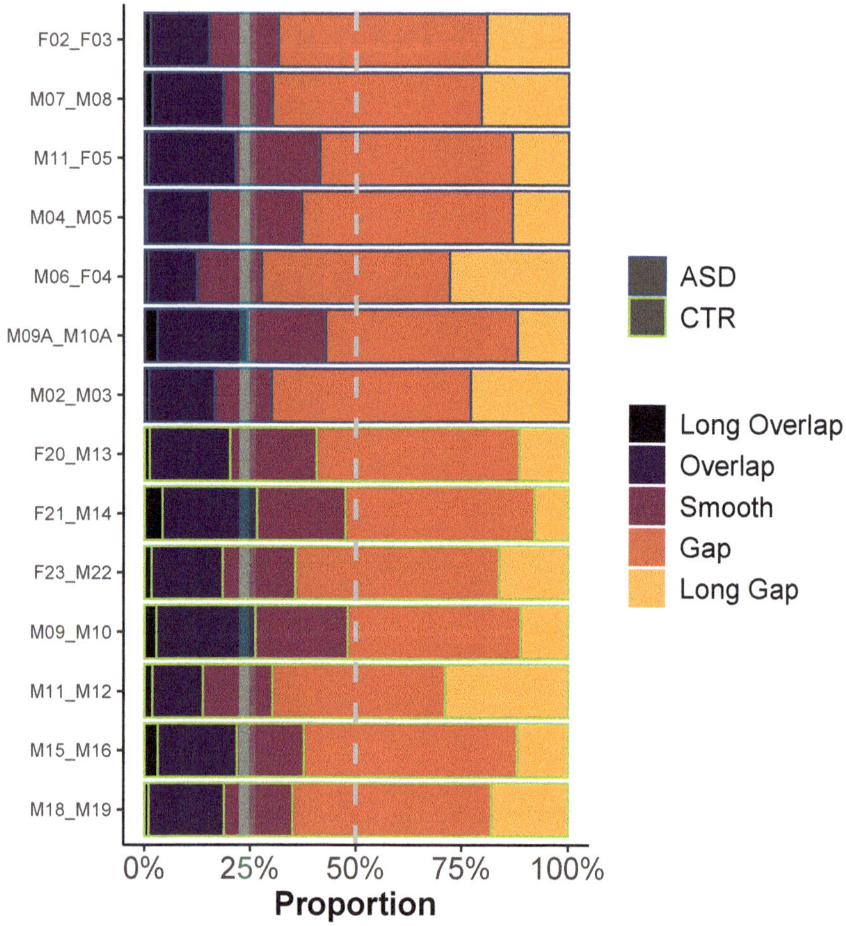

Figure B.2: Stacked bar charts by dyad showing proportions of different transition types. ASD dyads on top and outlined in blue, CTR group below and outlined in green. Transition proportions on the x-axis: long overlap transitions (FTO ≤-700 ms) in black, overlaps (FTO -699 ms – -100 ms) in dark purple, very short (*smooth*) transitions (FTO -99 – 99ms) in light purple, gaps (FTO 100 ms – 699 ms) in orange and long gaps (FTO ≤700 ms) in yellow.

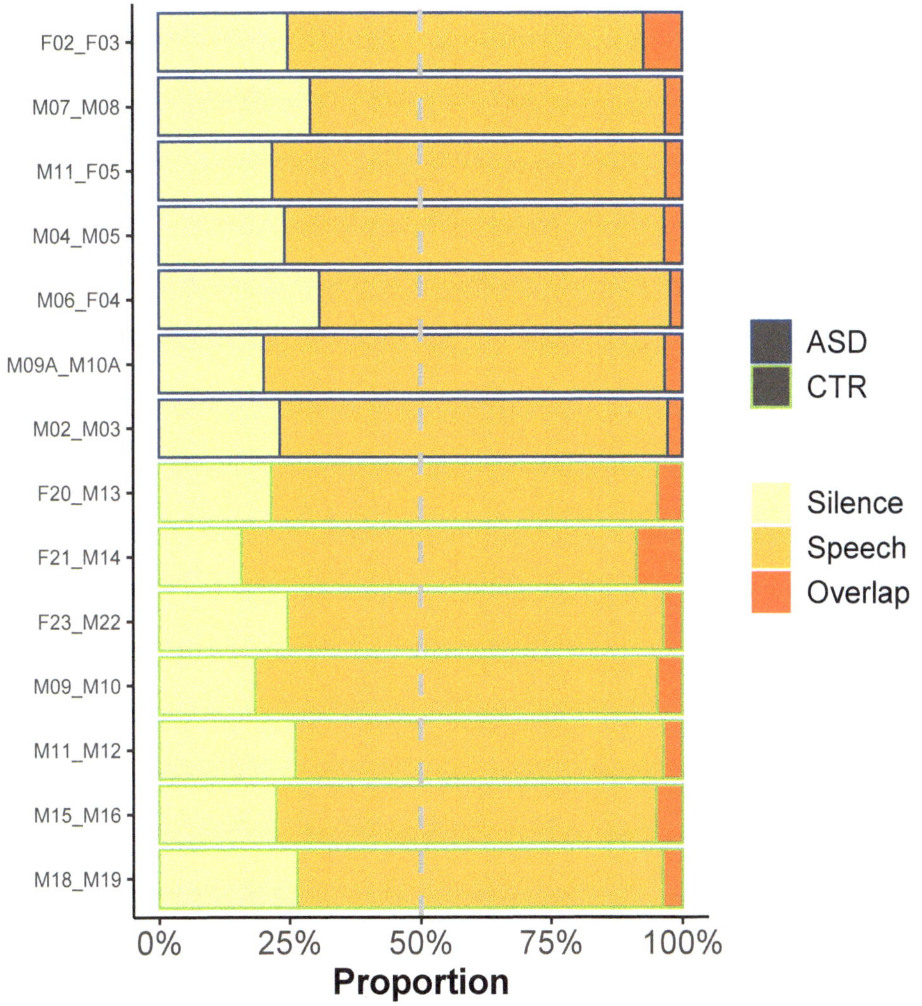

Figure B.3: ASD dyads on top and outlined in blue, CTR dyads below and outlined in green. Silence in beige, single-speaker speech in yellow, overlap in orange.

Appendix C: Backchannels and filled pauses

Figure C.1 shows proportions of backchannel type by speaker and group. Speakers from the same dyad are placed adjacent to each other. Table C.1 shows the ratio of rate of backchannels in the later stages of dialogue relative to rate of backchannels in the early stage of dialogue (before resolution of the first Mismatch). A ratio of 2, for instance, would indicate that a dyad produced twice as many backchannels per minute in the later stages compared to the early stage. Figure C.2 shows results from the categorical analysis of intonational realisation of filled pauses by speaker.

Table C.1: Ratios of backchannel rates in later stages relative to the early stage of dialogue.

Group	Dyad	Ratio
ASD	F02_F03	1.74
ASD	M07_M08	1.78
ASD	M11_F05	2.78
ASD	M04_M05	0.77
ASD	M06_F04	2.22
ASD	M09A_M10A	0.64
ASD	M02_M03	0.71
CTR	F20_M13	1.00
CTR	F21_M14	1.19
CTR	F23_M22	0.91
CTR	M09_M10	0.82
CTR	M11_M12	1.05
CTR	M15_M16	0.78
CTR	M18_M19	0.87

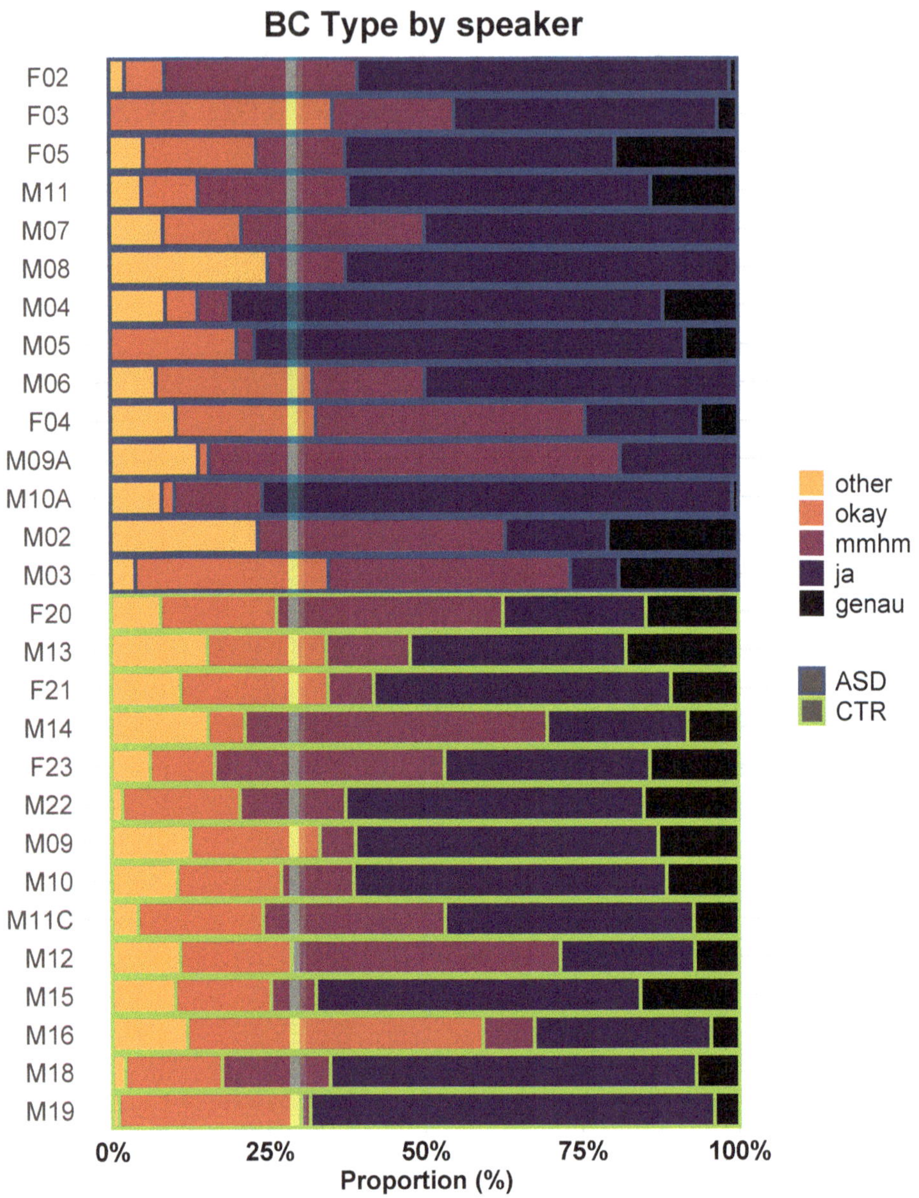

Figure C.1: Stacked bar charts by speaker showing proportions of different backchannel types. ASD group on top; CTR group below.

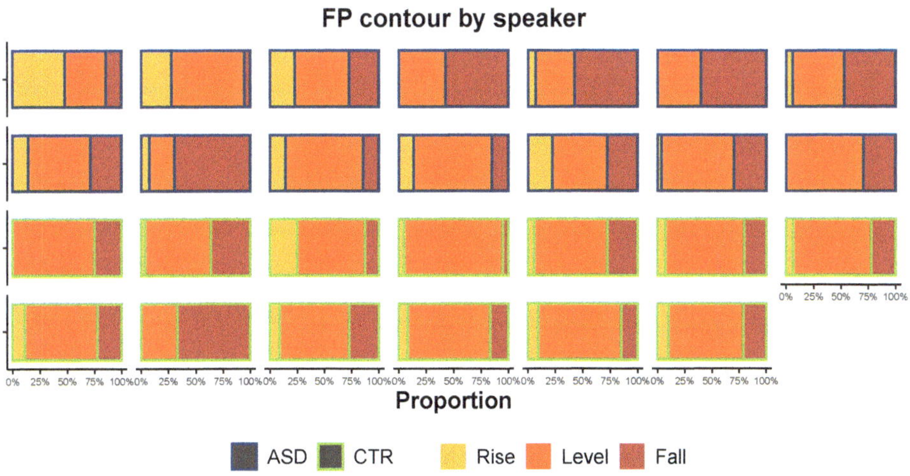

Figure C.2: Proportion of intonation contours produced on filled pauses, by speaker. ASD group in the two top rows and outlined in blue, CTR group on the two bottom rows and outlined in green. Rising contours in yellow, level contours in orange and falling contours in red. Level contours were defined as all tokens with a pitch difference in the range of ±1 semitone.

References

't Hart, Johan. 1981. Differential sensitivity to pitch distance, particularly in speech. *The Journal of the Acoustical Society of America* 69(3). 811–821.

Adell, Jordi, Antonio Bonafonte & David Escudero-Mancebo. 2010. Modelling filled pauses prosody to synthesise disfluent speech. In *Speech Prosody 2010-Fifth International Conference*.

Albert, Aviad. 2023. *A model of sonority based on pitch intelligibility*. Berlin, Germany: Language Science Press. DOI: 10.5281/zenodo.7837176.

Albert, Aviad, Francesco Cangemi, T. Mark Ellison & Martine Grice. 2020. *ProPer: PROsodic analysis with PERiodic energy*. DOI: 10.17605/OSF.IO/28EA5. (27 July, 2021).

Albert, Aviad, Francesco Cangemi & Martine Grice. 2018. Using periodic energy to enrich acoustic representations of pitch in speech: A demonstration. In *Proceedings Speech Prosody*, vol. 9, 13–16. Poznan, Poland.

Allaire, JJ, Yihui Xie, Christophe Dervieux, Jonathan McPherson, Javier Luraschi, Kevin Ushey, Aron Atkins, Hadley Wickham, Joe Cheng, Winston Chang & Richard Iannone. 2023. *Rmarkdown: Dynamic Documents for R*. Manual.

American Psychiatric Association. 2013. *Diagnostic and Statistical Manual of Mental Disorders (DSM-5®)*. American Psychiatric Pub.

Amrhein, Valentin, Sander Greenland & Blake McShane. 2019. Scientists rise up against statistical significance. *Nature* 567(7748). 305–307.

Anansiripinyo, Thanaporn & Chutamanee Onsuwan. 2019. Acoustic-phonetic characteristics of Thai filled pauses in monologues. In *The 9th Workshop on Disfluency in Spontaneous Speech*, 51–54.

Anderson, Anne, Miles Bader, Ellen Gurman Bard, Elizabeth Boyle, Gwyneth Doherty, Simon Garrod, Stephen Isard, Jacqueline Kowtko, Jan McAllister & Jim Miller. 1991. The HCRC map task corpus. *Language and Speech* 34(4). 351–366.

Anderson, Anne, Gillian Brown, Richard Shillcock & George Yule. 1984. *Teaching talk: Strategies for production and assessment*. Cambridge, UK: Cambridge University Press.

Anscombe, Francis J. 1973. Graphs in statistical analysis. *The American Statistician* 27(1). 17–21.

Ashwood, K. L., Nicola Gillan, Jamie Horder, Hannah Hayward, E. Woodhouse, Fiona Susan McEwen, James Findon, Hanna Eklund, Deborah Spain & C. E. Wilson. 2016. Predicting the diagnosis of autism in adults using the Autism-Spectrum Quotient (AQ) questionnaire. *Psychological Medicine* 46(12). 2595–2604.

Asperger, Hans. 1944. Die ‚Autistischen Psychopathen" im Kindesalter. *Archiv für Psychiatrie und Nervenkrankheiten* 117(1). 76–136. DOI: 10.1007/BF01837709.

Asperger, Hans & Uta Frith. 1991. 'Autistic psychopathy' in childhood. Translated and annotated by U. Frith. In Uta Frith (ed.), *Autism and Asperger Syndrome*, 37–92. Cambridge, UK: Cambridge University Press.

Auer, Peter. 2018. Gaze, addressee selection and turn-taking in three-party interaction. In Geert Brône & Bert Oben (eds.), *Eye-tracking in interaction: Studies on the role of eye gaze in dialogue*, vol. 197, 231. Amsterdam: John Benjamins Amsterdam.

Aust, Frederik & Marius Barth. 2022. *papaja: Prepare Reproducible APA Journal Articles with R Markdown.* Manual.

Aylett, Matthew & Alice Turk. 2004. The Smooth Signal Redundancy Hypothesis: A Functional Explanation for Relationships between Redundancy, Prosodic Prominence, and Duration in Spontaneous Speech. *Language and Speech* 47(1). 31–56. DOI: 10.1177/00238309040470010201.

Baltaxe, Christiane. 1984. Use of contrastive stress in normal, aphasic, and autistic children. *Journal of Speech, Language, and Hearing Research* 27(1). 97–105.

Baron-Cohen, Simon, Sally Wheelwright, Richard Skinner, Joanne Martin & Emma Clubley. 2001. The autism-spectrum quotient (AQ): Evidence from asperger syndrome/high-functioning autism, malesand females, scientists and mathematicians. *Journal of Autism and Developmental Disorders* 31(1). 5–17.

Barthel, Mathias, Antje S. Meyer & Stephen C. Levinson. 2017. Next speakers plan their turn early and speak after turn-final "go-signals". *Frontiers in Psychology* 8. 393.

Barthel, Mathias, Sebastian Sauppe, Stephen C. Levinson & Antje S. Meyer. 2016. The timing of utterance planning in task-oriented dialogue: Evidence from a novel list-completion paradigm. *Frontiers in Psychology* 7. 1858.

Beattie, Geoffrey W. 1979. Planning units in spontaneous speech: Some evidence from hesitation in speech and speaker gaze direction in conversation. *Linguistics* 17. 61–78.

Beckman, Mary E., Julia Bell Hirschberg & Stefanie Shattuck-Hufnagel. 2006. The original ToBI system and the evolution of the ToBI framework. In Sun-Ah Jun (ed.), *Prosodic typology: The phonology of intonation and phrasing*, 9–54. Oxford, UK: Oxford University Press.

Belz, Malte. 2021. *Die Phonetik von äh und ähm: Akustische Variation von Füllpartikeln im Deutschen.* Berlin, Germany: Springer Nature.

Belz, Malte & Uwe Reichel. 2015. Pitch characteristics of filled pauses. In *Proceedings of Disfluency in Spontaneous Speech (DiSS). The 7th Workshop on Disfluency in Spontaneous Speech.*

Belz, Malte & Jürgen Trouvain. 2019. Are 'Silent' Pauses Always Silent? In *19. International Congress of Phonetic Sciences (ICPhS)*, 2744–2748. Melbourne, Australia.

Beňuš, Štefan. 2009. Variability and stability in collaborative dialogues: Turn-taking and filled pauses. *Proceedings of the 10th INTERSPEECH conference.* 709–799.

Beňuš, Štefan, Agustín Gravano & Julia Bell Hirschberg. 2007. The prosody of backchannels in American English. In *Proceedings of 16th ICPhS.* Saarbrücken, Germany.

Betz, Simon, Robert Eklund & Petra Wagner. 2017. Prolongation in German. In *DiSS 2017 The 8th Workshop on Disfluency in Spontaneous Speech, KTH, Royal Institute of Technology, Stockholm, Sweden, 18–19 August 2017*, 13–16. KTH Royal Institute of Technology.

Bevacqua, Elisabetta, Sathish Pammi, Sylwia Julia Hyniewska, Marc Schröder & Catherine Pelachaud. 2010. Multimodal backchannels for embodied conversational agents. In *International Conference on Intelligent Virtual Agents*, 194–200. Springer.

Birdwhistell, Ray L. 1962. Critical moments in the psychiatric interview. In Thomas T. Tourlentes (ed.), *Research approaches to psychiatric problems*, 179–188. New York City, USA: Grune & Stratton.

Bishop, Dorothy. 2019. Rein in the four horsemen of irreproducibility. *Nature* 568(7753). 435–436.

Boersma & Weenink. 2021. *PRAAT: Doing phonetics by computer (Version 6.1.40).* http://www.praat.org/. (30 July, 2021).

Bögels, Sara & Stephen C. Levinson. 2017. The brain behind the response: Insights into turn-taking in conversation from neuroimaging. *Research on Language and Social Interaction* 50(1). 71–89.

Bögels, Sara & Francisco Torreira. 2015. Listeners use intonational phrase boundaries to project turn ends in spoken interaction. *Journal of Phonetics* 52. 46–57.

Bohus, Dan & Eric Horvitz. 2010. Facilitating multiparty dialog with gaze, gesture, and speech. In *International Conference on Multimodal Interfaces and the Workshop on Machine Learning for Multimodal Interaction*, 1–8.

Bolis, Dimitris, Joshua Balsters, Nicole Wenderoth, Cristina Becchio & Leonhard Schilbach. 2017. Beyond autism: Introducing the dialectical misattunement hypothesis and a Bayesian account of Intersubjectivity. *Psychopathology* 50(6). 355–372. DOI: 10.1159/000484353.

Boo, Cynthia, Nora Alpers-Leon, Nancy McIntyre, Peter Mundy & Letitia Naigles. 2022. Conversation during a virtual reality task reveals new structural language profiles of children with ASD, ADHD, and comorbid symptoms of both. *Journal of Autism and Developmental Disorders* 52(7). 2970–2983. DOI: 10.1007/s10803-021-05175-6.

Botha, Monique, Jacqueline Hanlon & Gemma Louise Williams. 2021. Does language matter? Identity-first versus person-first language use in autism research: A response to Vivanti. *Journal of Autism and Developmental Disorders* 53. 870–878.

Bottema-Beutel, Kristen, Steven K. Kapp, Jessica Nina Lester, Noah J. Sasson & Brittany N. Hand. 2021. Avoiding ableist language: Suggestions for autism researchers. *Autism in Adulthood* 3(1). 18–29.

Bradlow, Ann R., Midam Kim & Michael Blasingame. 2017. Language-independent talker-specificity in first-language and second-language speech production by bilingual talkers: L1 speaking rate predicts L2 speaking rate. *The Journal of the Acoustical Society of America* 141(2). 886–899.

Breitholtz, Ellen, Robin Cooper, Christine Howes & Mary Lavelle. 2021. Reasoning in multiparty dialogue involving patients with schizophrenia. In M. Amblard, M. Musiol & M. Rebuschi (eds.), *(In-)Coherence of discourse: Formal and conceptual issues of language*, 43–63. Cham, Switzerland: Springer.

Brône, Geert, Bert Oben, Annelies Jehoul, Jelena Vranjes & Kurt Feyaerts. 2017. Eye gaze and viewpoint in multimodal interaction management. *Cognitive Linguistics* 28(3). 449–483.

Bruggeman, Anna, Francesco Cangemi, Simon Wehrle, Dina El Zarka & Martine Grice. 2017. Unifying speaker variability with the Tonal Centre of Gravity. *Proceedings of the Conference on Phonetics & Phonology in German-speaking countries (2018).* 21–24.

Brysbaert, Marc. 2020. Power considerations in bilingualism research: Time to step up our game. *Bilingualism: Language and Cognition* 24. 1–6.

Bürkner, Paul-Christian. 2017. Brms: An R package for Bayesian multilevel models using Stan. *Journal of Statistical Software* 80(1). 1–28.

Campbell, Nick. 2007. Approaches to conversational speech rhythm: Speech activity in two-person telephone dialogues. In *Proc XVIth International Congress of the Phonetic Sciences, Saarbrucken, Germany*, 343–348.

Cangemi, Francesco. 2015. *Mausmooth.* Retrievable online at http://phonetik.phil-fak. uni-koeln.de/fcangemi.html.

Cangemi, Francesco, Aviad Albert & Martine Grice. 2019. Modelling intonation: Beyond segments and tonal targets. In *Proceedings of the 19th International Congress of Phonetic Sciences, Melbourne, Australia.*

Cangemi, Francesco, Dina El Zarka, Simon Wehrle, Stefan Baumann & Martine Grice. 2016. Speaker-specific intonational marking of narrow focus in Egyptian Arabic. In *Proceedings of Speech Prosody 2016*, 335–339. Boston, USA.

Cangemi, Francesco & Martine Grice. 2016. The importance of a distributional approach to categoriality in autosegmental-metrical accounts of intonation. *Laboratory Phonology: Journal of the Association for Laboratory Phonology* 7(1). DOI: 10.5334/labphon.28.

Cangemi, Francesco, Martine Grice, Alicia Janz, Valeria Lucarini, Malin Spaniol & Kai Vogeley. 2023. Content-free speech activity records: Interviews with people with schizophrenia. *Language Resources and Evaluation.* DOI: 10.1007/s10579-023-09666-z.

Cangemi, Francesco, Martina Krüger & Martine Grice. 2015. Listener-specific perception of speaker-specific production in intonation. In Susanne Fuchs, Daniel Pape, Caterina Petrone & Pascal Perrier (eds.), *Individual differences in speech production and perception*, 123–145. Frankfurt, Germany: Peter Lang.

Cannon, Jonathan, Amanda M. O'Brien, Lindsay Bungert & Pawan Sinha. 2021. Prediction in autism spectrum disorder: A systematic review of empirical evidence. *Autism Research* 14(4). 604–630. DOI: 10.1002/aur.2482.

Carletta, Jean, Amy Isard, Stephen Isard, Jacqueline C. Kowtko, Gwyneth Doherty-Sneddon & Anne H. Anderson. 1997. The reliability of a dialogue structure coding scheme. *Computational Linguistics* 23. 13–31.

Carpenter, Bob, Andrew Gelman, Matthew D. Hoffman, Daniel Lee, Ben Goodrich, Michael Betancourt, Marcus A. Brubaker, Jiqiang Guo, Peter Li & Allen Riddell. 2017. Stan: A probabilistic programming language. *Journal of Statistical Software* 76(1). 1–32.

Casillas, Marisa, Susan C. Bobb & Eve V. Clark. 2016. Turn taking, timing, and planning in early language acquisition. *Journal of Child Language* 43. 1310–1337.

Caspers, Johanneke. 2000. Melodic characteristics of backchannels in Dutch Map Task dialogues. In *Proceedings of the 6th International Conference on Spoken Language Processing*, 611–614.

Celce-Murcia, Marianne, Donna M. Brinton & Janet M. Goodwin. 1996. *Teaching pronunciation: A reference for teachers of English to speakers of other languages.* Cambridge, UK: Cambridge University Press.

Chan, Kary K. L. & Carol K. S. To. 2016. Do individuals with high-functioning autism who speak a tone language show intonation deficits? *Journal of Autism and Developmental Disorders* 46(5). 1784–1792.

Chasson, Gregory & S. R. Jarosiewicz. 2014. Social competence impairments in autism spectrum disorders. In Vinood B. Patel, Victor R. Preedy & Colin R. Martin (eds.), *Comprehensive guide to autism*, 1099–1108. New York City, USA: Springer.

Cho, Hyongsil & Daniel Hirst. 2006. The contribution of silent pauses to the perception of prosodic boundaries in Korean read speech. *Proceedings of Speech Prosody 2006*.

Choi, Jieun & Yoonkyoung Lee. 2013. Conversational Turn-Taking and Topic Manipulation Skills of Children with High-Functioning Autism Spectrum Disorders. *Communication Sciences & Disorders* 18(1). 12–23. DOI: 10.12963/csd.13002.

Christensen, Deborah L., Kim Van Naarden Braun, Jon Baio, Deborah Bilder, Jane Charles, John N. Constantino, Julie Daniels, Maureen S. Durkin, Robert T. Fitzgerald & Margaret Kurzius-Spencer. 2018. Prevalence and characteristics of autism spectrum disorder among children aged 8 Years: Autism and developmental disabilities monitoring network, 11 sites, United States, 2012. *MMWR Surveillance Summaries* 65(13). 1.

Christiansen, Morten H. & Nick Chater. 2016. *Creating language: Integrating evolution, acquisition, and processing*. Boston, USA: MIT Press.

Clark, Herbert H. & Jean E. Fox Tree. 2002. Using uh and um in spontaneous speaking. *Cognition* 84(1). 73–111. DOI: 10.1016/S0010-0277(02)00017-3.

Clark, Herbert H. & Edward F. Schaefer. 1989. Contributing to discourse. *Cognitive Science* 13(2). 259–294.

Cohen, Jacob. 1988. *Statistical power analysis for the behavioral sciences*. New York, USA: Routledge.

Cooper, William E & John M Sorensen. 1981. *Fundamental frequency in sentence production*. Berlin, Germany: Springer.

Coretta, Stefano et al. 2023. Multidimensional signals and analytic flexibility: Estimating degrees of freedom in human-speech analyses. *Advances in Methods and Practices in Psychological Science* 6(3). 25152459231162567. DOI: 10.1177/25152459231162567.

Corley, Martin & Robert J. Hartsuiker. 2003. Hesitation in speech can... um... help a listener understand. In *Proceedings of the Annual Meeting of the Cognitive Science Society*, vol. 25.

Council of Europe. 2001. *Common European Framework of Reference for Languages: Learning, teaching, assessment*. Cambridge: Cambridge University Press.

Couper-Kuhlen, Elizabeth & Dagmar Barth-Weingarten. 2011. A system for transcribing talk-in-interaction: GAT 2: English translation and adaptation of Selting, Margret et al.: Gesprächsanalytisches Transkriptionssystem 2. *Gesprächsforschung* 12. 1–51.

Crompton, Catherine J., Martha Sharp, Harriet Axbey, Sue Fletcher-Watson, Emma G. Flynn & Danielle Ropar. 2020. Neurotype-matching, but not being autistic, influences self and observer ratings of interpersonal rapport. *Frontiers in Psychology* 11. DOI: 10.3389/fpsyg.2020.586171/full.

Cutrone, Pino. 2005. A case study examining backchannels in conversations between Japanese–British dyads. *Multilingua* 24(3). 237–274. DOI: 10.1515/mult.2005.24.3.237.

Cutrone, Pino. 2014. A cross-cultural examination of the backchannel behavior of Japanese and Americans: Considerations for Japanese EFL learners. *Intercultural Pragmatics* 11(1). 83–120.

D'Imperio, Mariapaola, Martine Grice & Francesco Cangemi. 2016. Advancing prosodic transcription: Special collection. *Journal of the Association for Laboratory Phonology* 7.

Davis, Rachael & Catherine J. Crompton. 2021. What do new findings about social interaction in autistic adults mean for neurodevelopmental research? *Perspectives on Psychological Science* 16(3). 649–653. DOI: 10.1177/1745691620958010.

De Jong, Nivja H. & Hans R. Bosker. 2013. Choosing a threshold for silent pauses to measure second language fluency. In *The 6th Workshop on Disfluency in Spontaneous Speech (DISS)*, 17–20.

De Marchena, A., E. S. Kim, A. Bagdasarov, J. Parish-Morris, B. B. Maddox, E. S. Brodkin & R. T. Schultz. 2019. Atypicalities of gesture form and function in autistic adults. *Journal of Autism and Developmental Disorders* 49(4). 1438–1454.

De Moraes, João Antônio. 1998. Intonation in Brazilian Portuguese. In Daniel Hirst & Albert Di Cristo (eds.), *Intonation systems. A survey of twenty languages*, 179–194. Cambridge: Cambridge University Press, Cambridge.

De Ruiter, Jan-Peter, Holger Mitterer & Nick J. Enfield. 2006. Projecting the end of a speaker's turn: A cognitive cornerstone of conversation. *Language* 82(3). 515–535.

De Ruiter, Laura E. 2015. Information status marking in spontaneous vs. Read speech in story-telling tasks–Evidence from intonation analysis using GToBI. *Journal of Phonetics* 48. 29–44.

DePape, Anne-Marie R., Aoju Chen, Geoffrey BC Hall & Laurel J. Trainor. 2012. Use of prosody and information structure in high functioning adults with autism in relation to language ability. *Frontiers in Psychology* 3. 72.

Derwing, Tracey M. & Murray J. Munro. 2009. Putting accent in its place: Rethinking obstacles to communication. *Language Teaching* 42(4). 476–490.

DeVito, Nicholas J. & Ben Goldacre. 2019. Catalogue of bias: Publication bias. *BMJ Evidence-Based Medicine* 24(2). 53–54.

Di Napoli, Jessica. 2020. Filled pauses and prolongations in Roman Italian task-oriented dialogue. In *Laughter and Other Non-Verbal Vocalisations Workshop: Proceedings (2020)*, 24–27.

Dideriksen, Christina, Riccardo Fusaroli, Kristian Tylén, Mark Dingemanse & Morten H. Christiansen. 2019. Contextualizing conversational strategies: Backchannel, repair and linguistic alignment in spontaneous and task-oriented conversations. In *CogSci'19*, 261–267. Cognitive Science Society.

Diehl, Joshua J., Duane Watson, Loisa Bennetto, Joyce McDonough & Christine Gunlogson. 2009. An acoustic analysis of prosody in high-functioning autism. *Applied Psycholinguistics* 30(3). 385.

Dienes, Zoltan. 2011. Bayesian versus orthodox statistics: Which side are you on? *Perspectives on Psychological Science* 6(3). 274–290.

Dingemanse, Mark & Andreas Liesenfeld. 2022. From text to talk: Harnessing conversational corpora for humane and diversity-aware language technology. In *Proceedings of the 60th Annual Meeting of the Association for Computational Linguistics (Volume 1: Long Papers)*. Dublin, Ireland.

Dingemanse, Mark, Andreas Liesenfeld, Marlou Rasenberg, Saul Albert, Felix K. Ameka, Abeba Birhane, Dimitris Bolis, Justine Cassell, Rebecca Clift, Elena Cuffari, Hanne De Jaegher, Catarina Dutilh Novaes, N. J. Enfield, Riccardo Fusaroli, Eleni Gregoromichelaki, Edwin Hutchins, Ivana Konvalinka, Damian Milton, Joanna Rączaszek-Leonardi, Vasudevi Reddy, Federico Rossano, David Schlangen, Johanna Seibt, Elizabeth Stokoe, Lucy Suchman, Cordula Vesper, Thalia Wheatley & Martina Wiltschko. 2023. Beyond single-mindedness: A figure-ground reversal for the Cognitive Sciences. *Cognitive Science* 47(1). e13230. DOI: 10.1111/cogs.13230.

Dunn, Dana S. & Erin E. Andrews. 2015. Person-first and identity-first language: Developing psychologists' cultural competence using disability language. *American Psychologist* 70(3). 255.

Durand, Jacques. 2010. Le français méridional: éléments de synthèse. In Sylvan Detey, Jacques Durand, Bernard Laks & Chantal Lyche (eds.), *Les variétés du français parlé dans l'espace francophone: Ressources pour l'enseignement*, vol. 36, 243–262. Paris: Ophrys.

Eager, Christopher & Joseph Roy. 2017. Mixed effects models are sometimes terrible. *arXiv preprint arXiv:1701.04858.*

Easterbrook, Phillipa J., Ramana Gopalan, J. A. Berlin & David R. Matthews. 1991. Publication bias in clinical research. *The Lancet* 337(8746). 867–872.
Edelson, L., R. Grossman & H. Tager-Flusberg. 2007. Emotional prosody in children and adolescents with autism. In *Poster session presented at the Annual International Meeting for Autism Research, Seattle, WA.*
Ehlich, Konrad. 1986. *Interjektionen*, vol. 111. Tubingen, Germany: Niemeyer.
Eigsti, Inge-Marie, Loisa Bennetto & Mamta B. Dadlani. 2007. Beyond pragmatics: Morphosyntactic development in autism. *Journal of Autism and Developmental Disorders* 37(6). 1007–1023.
Elsabbagh, Mayada, Gauri Divan, Yun-Joo Koh, Young Shin Kim, Shuaib Kauchali, Carlos Marcín, Cecilia Montiel-Nava, Vikram Patel, Cristiane S. Paula & Chongying Wang. 2012. Global prevalence of autism and other pervasive developmental disorders. *Autism Research* 5(3). 160–179.
Engelhardt, Paul E., Oliver Alfridijanta, Mhairi E. G. McMullon & Martin Corley. 2017. Speaker-versus listener-oriented disfluency: A re-examination of arguments and assumptions from Autism Spectrum Disorder. *Journal of Autism and Developmental Disorders* 47(9). 2885–2898. DOI: 10.1007/s10803-017-3215-0.
Erard, Michael. 2008. *Um...: Slips, stumbles, and verbal blunders, and what they mean.* New York City, USA: Anchor.
Evans, Nicholas & Stephen C. Levinson. 2009. The myth of language universals: Language diversity and its importance for cognitive science. *Behavioral and Brain Sciences* 32(5). 429–448.
Fay, Warren H. & Adriana Luce Schuler. 1980. *Emerging language in autistic children.* London: Edward Arnold.
Feldstein, Stanley, Mary Konstantareas, Joel Oxman & Christopher D. Webster. 1982. The chronography of interactions with autistic speakers: An initial report. *Journal of Communication Disorders* 15(6). 451–460.
Fischer, Kerstin. 2000. Discourse particles, turn-taking, and the semantics-pragmatics interface. *Revue de Sémantique et Pragmatique* 8. 111–132.
Fischer, Kerstin. 2013. *From cognitive semantics to lexical pragmatics.* Berlin, Germany: De Gruyter Mouton.
Fosnot, Susan Meyers & Sun-Ah Jun. 1999. Prosodic characteristics in children with stuttering or autism during reading and imitation. In *Proceedings of the 14th International Congress of Phonetic Sciences*, 1925–1928. San Francisco, USA.
Fox Tree, Jean E. 2001. Listeners' uses of um and uh in speech comprehension. *Memory & Cognition* 29(2). 320–326.
Fox Tree, Jean E. 2002. Interpreting pauses and ums at turn exchanges. *Discourse Processes* 34(1). 37–55.

Franke, Michael & Timo B. Roettger. 2019. Bayesian regression modeling (for factorial designs): A tutorial. *Preprint (psyarxiv) retrievable from https://psyarxiv.com/cdxv3.*

Frazier, Thomas W., Eric A. Youngstrom, Leslie Speer, Rebecca Embacher, Paul Law, John Constantino, Robert L. Findling, Antonio Y. Hardan & Charis Eng. 2012. Validation of proposed DSM-5 criteria for autism spectrum disorder. *Journal of the American Academy of Child & Adolescent Psychiatry* 51(1). 28–40.

Fries, Charles Carpenter. 1952. *The structure of English.* New York: Harcourt, Brace and Co.

Frith, Uta. 2003. *Autism: Explaining the enigma.* Oxford, UK: Blackwell Publishing.

Fröhlich, Marlen, Paul Kuchenbuch, Gudrun Müller, Barbara Fruth, Takeshi Furuichi, Roman M. Wittig & Simone Pika. 2016. Unpeeling the layers of language: Bonobos and chimpanzees engage in cooperative turn-taking sequences. *Scientific Reports* 6(1). 1–14.

Frota, Sónia. 2016. Surface and Structure: Transcribing intonation within and across languages. *Laboratory Phonology* 7(1). 1–19.

Fruehwald, Josef. 2016. Filled pause choice as a sociolinguistic variable. *University of Pennsylvania Working Papers in Linguistics* 22(2). 41–49.

Fuchs, Susanne, Caterina Petrone, Amélie Rochet-Capellan, Uwe D. Reichel & Laura L. Koenig. 2015. Assessing respiratory contributions to f0 declination in German across varying speech tasks and respiratory demands. *Journal of Phonetics* 52. 35–45.

Fujie, Shinya, Kenta Fukushima & Tetsunori Kobayashi. 2004. A conversation robot with back-channel feedback function based on linguistic and nonlinguistic information. In *Proc. ICARA Int. Conference on Autonomous Robots and Agents*, 379–384.

Fujimoto, Donna T. 2009. Listener responses in interaction: A case for abandoning the term, backchannel. *Journal of Osaka Jogakuin College* 37. 35–54.

Gabry, Jonah & Tristan Mahr. 2022. *Bayesplot: Plotting for Bayesian models.*

Galaczi, Evelina D. 2014. Interactional competence across proficiency levels: How do learners manage interaction in paired speaking tests? *Applied Linguistics* 35(5). 553–574.

Garnier, Simon, Ross, Noam, Rudis, Robert, Camargo, Antônio Pedro, Sciaini, Marco, Scherer & Cédric. 2023. *Viridis(Lite) - colorblind-friendly color maps for R.* Manual. DOI: 10.5281/zenodo.4679424.

Garvey, Catherine & Ginger Berninger. 1981. Timing and turn taking in children's conversations. *Discourse Processes* 4(1). 27–57.

Gelman, Andrew, Aki Vehtari, Daniel Simpson, Charles C. Margossian, Bob Carpenter, Yuling Yao, Lauren Kennedy, Jonah Gabry, Paul-Christian Bürkner & Martin Modrák. 2020. Bayesian Workflow. *arXiv preprint arXiv:2011.01808.*

Gernsbacher, Morton Ann. 2017. Editorial perspective: The use of person-first language in scholarly writing May accentuate stigma. *Journal of Child Psychology and Psychiatry* 58(7). 859–861.

Gernsbacher, Morton Ann, Emily M. Morson & Elizabeth J. Grace. 2016. Language and Speech in Autism. *Annual Review of Linguistics* 2(1). 413–425. DOI: 10.1146/annurev-linguistics-030514-124824.

Gernsbacher, Morton Ann, Eve A. Sauer, Heather M. Geye, Emily K. Schweigert & H. Hill Goldsmith. 2008. Infant and toddler oral-and manual-motor skills predict later speech fluency in autism. *Journal of Child Psychology and Psychiatry* 49(1). 43–50.

Gervais, Matthew & David Sloan Wilson. 2005. The evolution and functions of laughter and Humor: A synthetic approach. *The Quarterly Review of Biology* 80(4). 395–430.

Gleitman, Lila R., David January, Rebecca Nappa & John C. Trueswell. 2007. On the give and take between event apprehension and utterance formulation. *Journal of Memory and Language* 57(4). 544–569.

Goldberg, Adele E. & Kirsten Abbot-Smith. 2021. The constructionist approach offers a useful lens on language learning in autistic individuals: Response to Kissine. *Language* 97(3). e169–e183. DOI: 10.1353/lan.2021.0035.

Goldfarb, William, Nathan Goldfarb, Patricia Braunstein & Hannah Scholl. 1972. Speech and language faults of schizophrenic children. *Journal of Autism and Childhood Schizophrenia* 2(3). 219–233.

Goldman-Eisler, Frieda. 1968. *Psycholinguistics: Experiments in spontaneous speech.* New York: Academic Press.

Gorman, Kyle, Lindsay Olson, Alison Presmanes Hill, Rebecca Lunsford, Peter A. Heeman & Jan PH van Santen. 2016. Uh and um in children with autism spectrum disorders or language impairment. *Autism Research* 9(8). 854–865.

Graham, Calbert. 2014. Fundamental frequency range in Japanese and English: The case of simultaneous bilinguals. *Phonetica* 71(4). 271–295.

Gratier, Maya, Emmanuel Devouche, Bahia Guellai, Rubia Infanti, Ebru Yilmaz & Erika Parlato-Oliveira. 2015. Early development of turn-taking in vocal interaction between mothers and infants. *Frontiers in Psychology* 6(1167). 236–245.

Green, Hila. 2009. Intonation in Hebrew-speaking children with high functioning autism. *Asia Pacific Journal of Speech, Language and Hearing* 12(2). 187–198.

Green, Hila & Yishai Tobin. 2008. Intonation in Hebrew speaking children with highfunctioning autism: A case study. In *Proceedings of the fourth Conference on Speech Prosody SP2008*, 237–240. Campinas, Brazil.

Green, Hila & Yishai Tobin. 2009. Prosodic analysis is difficult... but worth it: A study in high functioning autism. *International Journal of Speech-Language Pathology* 11(4). 308–315.

Grice, Martine, Simon Ritter, Henrik Niemann & Timo B. Roettger. 2017. Integrating the discreteness and continuity of intonational categories. *Journal of Phonetics* 64. 90–107. DOI: 10.1016/j.wocn.2017.03.003.

Grice, Martine & Michelina Savino. 2003. Map tasks in Italian: Asking questions about given, accessible and new information. *Catalan Journal of Linguistics* 2. 153–180.

Grice, Martine, Michelina Savino & Mario Refice. 1997. The intonation of questions in Bari Italian: Do speakers replicate their spontaneous speech when reading. *Phonus* 3. 1–7.

Grice, Martine, Michelina Savino & Timo B. Roettger. 2018. Word final Schwa is driven by intonation—The case of Bari Italian. *The Journal of the Acoustical Society of America* 143(4). 2474–2486.

Grice, Martine, Simon Wehrle, Martina Krüger, Malin Spaniol, Francesco Cangemi & Kai Vogeley. 2023. Linguistic Prosody in Autism Spectrum Disorder—An Overview. *Language and Linguistics Compass*. DOI: 10.1111/lnc3.12498.

Grieve, Jack. 2021. Observation, experimentation, and replication in linguistics. *Linguistics*. DOI: 10.1515/ling-2021-0094.

Griffin, Zenzi M. & Kathryn Bock. 2000. What the eyes say about speaking. *Psychological Science* 11(4). 274–279.

Gussenhoven, Carlos & Antonius Clemens Maria Rietveld. 1988. Fundamental frequency declination in Dutch: Testing three hypotheses. *Journal of Phonetics* 16(3). 355–369.

Ha, Kieu-Phuong. 2012. *Prosody in Vietnamese: Intonational form and function of short utterances in conversation*. Canberra, Australia: The Australian National University - Asia-Pacific Linguistics (SEAMLES).

Ha, Kieu-Phuong, Samuel Ebner & Martine Grice. 2016. Speech prosody and possible misunderstandings in intercultural talk: A study of listener behaviour in Standard Vietnamese and German dialogues. In *Proceedings of Speech Prosody 2016*, 801–805. Boston, USA.

Ha, Kieu-Phuong & Martine Grice. 2010. Modelling the interaction of intonation and lexical tone in Vietnamese. In *Speech Prosody 2010*. Chicago, USA.

Hall, Peter & James S. Marron. 1991. Local Minima in Cross-Validation Functions. *Journal of the Royal Statistical Society: Series B (Methodological)* 53(1). 245–252. DOI: 10.1111/j.2517-6161.1991.tb01822.x.

Hanulová, Jana, Douglas J. Davidson & Peter Indefrey. 2011. Where does the delay in L2 picture naming come from? Psycholinguistic and neurocognitive evidence on second language word production. *Language and Cognitive Processes* 26(7). 902–934.

Happé, Francesca. 1995. Understanding minds and metaphors: Insights from the study of figurative language in autism. *Metaphor and Symbol* 10(4). 275–295.

Happé, Francesca, Jacqueline Briskman & Uta Frith. 2001. Exploring the cognitive phenotype of autism: Weak "Central coherence" in parents and siblings of children with autism: I. Experimental tests. *Journal of Child Psychology and Psychiatry* 42(3). 299–307.

Hawkins, Sarah, Ian Cross & Richard Ogden. 2013. Communicative interaction in spontaneous music and speech. In Martin Orwin, Christine Howes & Ruth Kempson (eds.), *Music, language and interaction*, 285–329. London, UK: College Publications.

Head, Megan L., Luke Holman, Rob Lanfear, Andrew T. Kahn & Michael D. Jennions. 2015. The extent and consequences of p-hacking in science. *PLoS Biology* 13(3). e1002106.

Heeman, Peter A., Rebecca Lunsford, Ethan Selfridge, Lois M. Black & Jan Van Santen. 2010. Autism and interactional aspects of dialogue. In *Proceedings of the SIGDIAL 2010 Conference*, 249–252.

Heldner, Mattias & Jens Edlund. 2010. Pauses, gaps and overlaps in conversations. *Journal of Phonetics* 38(4). 555–568.

Heldner, Mattias, Jens Edlund, Anna Hjalmarsson & Kornel Laskowski. 2011. Very short utterances and timing in turn-taking. In *Twelfth Annual Conference of the International Speech Communication Association*.

Hillary, Alyssa. 2020. Neurodiversity and cross-cultural communication. In H. Bertilsdotter Rosqvist, N. Chown & A Stenning (eds.), *Neurodiversity Studies*, 91–107. London, UK: Routledge.

Hind, Anthony. 1999. Regularity, melodicity, and stereotyping, in French and English intonation systems. In *14th International Congress of Phonetic Sciences*. San Francisco, USA.

Hind, Anthony. 2002. Metrical patterns and melodicity in English contrasted with French. In *Speech Prosody 2002*. Aix-en-Provence, France.

Hirst, Daniel & Albert Di Cristo. 1998. *Intonation systems: A survey of twenty languages*. Cambridge, UK: Cambridge University Press.

Hjalmarsson, Anna & Catharine Oertel. 2012. Gaze direction as a back-channel inviting cue in dialogue. In *IVA 2012 Workshop on Realtime Conversational Virtual Agents*, vol. 9.

Hodges-Simeon, Carolyn R., Steven JC Gaulin & David A. Puts. 2010. Different vocal parameters predict perceptions of dominance and attractiveness. *Human Nature* 21(4). 406–427.

Holler, Judith, Kobin H. Kendrick & Stephen C. Levinson. 2018. Processing language in face-to-face conversation: Questions with gestures get faster responses. *Psychonomic Bulletin & Review* 25(5). 1900–1908.

Holmes, Janet. 2013. *An introduction to sociolinguistics*. London, UK: Routledge.

Howes, Christine, Mary Lavelle, Patrick GT Healey, Julian Hough & Rosemarie McCabe. 2017. Disfluencies in dialogues with patients with schizophrenia. In *Proc. Of the 39th Annual Meeting of the Cognitive Science Society*. London, UK.

Hualde, José Ignacio & Pilar Prieto. 2016. Towards an international prosodic alphabet (IPrA). *Laboratory Phonology* 7(1). DOI: 10.5334/labphon.11.

Hubbard, Kathleen & Doris A. Trauner. 2007. Intonation and emotion in autistic spectrum disorders. *Journal of Psycholinguistic Research* 36(2). 159–173.

Hudenko, William J., Wendy Stone & Jo-Anne Bachorowski. 2009. Laughter differs in children with autism: An acoustic analysis of laughs produced by children with and without the disorder. *Journal of Autism and Developmental Disorders* 39(10). 1392–1400.

Hull, Laura, K. V. Petrides, Carrie Allison, Paula Smith, Simon Baron-Cohen, Meng-Chuan Lai & William Mandy. 2017. "Putting on my best normal": Social camouflaging in adults with autism spectrum conditions. *Journal of Autism and Developmental Disorders* 47(8). 2519–2534.

Irvine, Christina A., Inge-Marie Eigsti & Deborah A. Fein. 2016. Uh, um, and autism: Filler disfluencies as pragmatic markers in adolescents with optimal outcomes from autism spectrum disorder. *Journal of Autism and Developmental Disorders* 46(3). 1061–1070.

Janz, Alicia. 2019. *Turn-transitions on the spectrum: The conversational effect of unexpectedness*. Cologne, Germany: University of Cologne. (BA Thesis).

Janz, Alicia. 2022. *Navigating common ground using feedback in conversation- A phonetic analysis*. Cologne, Germany: University of Cologne. (MA thesis).

Jefferson, Gail. 1984. Notes on a systematic deployment of the acknowledgement tokens "yeah"; and "mm hm". *Paper in Linguistics* 17(2). 197–216.

John, Leslie K., George Loewenstein & Drazen Prelec. 2012. Measuring the prevalence of questionable research practices with incentives for truth telling. *Psychological Science* 23(5). 524–532. DOI: 10.1177/0956797611430953.

Jones, Rebekah, Emily R Zane & Ruth B Grossman. 2022. Like, it's important: The frequency and use of the discourse marker like in older autistic children. *Autism & Developmental Language Impairments* 7. 23969415221129132. DOI: 10.1177/23969415221129132.

Jongman, Allard, Zhen Qin, Jie Zhang & Joan A. Sereno. 2017. Just noticeable differences for pitch direction, height, and slope for Mandarin and English listeners. *The Journal of the Acoustical Society of America* 142(2). EL163–EL169.

Jun, Sun-Ah. 2012. Prosodic typology revisited: Adding macro-rhythm. In *Speech Prosody 2012*. Shanghai, China.

Jun, Sun-Ah. 2014. Prosodic typology: By prominence type, word prosody, and macro-rhythm. In Sun-Ah Jun (ed.), *Prosodic typology II*, 520–539. Oxford, UK: Oxford University Press.

Jurafsky, Dan, Elizabeth Shriberg, Barbara Fox & Traci Curl. 1998. Lexical, prosodic, and syntactic cues for dialog acts. In *Workshop on Discourse Relations and Discourse Markers*, 114–120.

Kaland, Constantijn. 2022. Bending the string: Intonation contour length as a correlate of macro-rhythm. *Proceedings of Interspeech 2022*. 5233–5237.

Kaland, Constantijn, Marc Swerts & Emiel Krahmer. 2013. Accounting for the listener: Comparing the production of contrastive intonation in typically-developing speakers and speakers with autism. *The Journal of the Acoustical Society of America* 134(3). 2182–2196.

Kanner, Leo. 1943. Autistic disturbances of affective contact. *Nervous Child* 2(3). 217–250.

Kay, Matthew. 2023. *tidybayes: Tidy data and geoms for Bayesian models*. Manual. DOI: 10.5281/zenodo.1308151.

Keltner, Dacher & George A. Bonanno. 1997. A study of laughter and dissociation: Distinct correlates of laughter and smiling during bereavement. *Journal of Personality and Social Psychology* 73(4). 687.

Kendon, Adam. 1967. Some functions of gaze-direction in social interaction. *Acta Psychologica* 26. 22–63. DOI: 10.1016/0001-6918(67)90005-4.

Kendrick, Kobin H. 2015. The intersection of turn-taking and repair: The timing of other-initiations of repair in conversation. *Frontiers in Psychology* 6(250). 10–3389.

Kendrick, Kobin H. & Francisco Torreira. 2015. The timing and construction of preference: A quantitative study. *Discourse Processes* 52(4). 255–289.

Kerr, Norbert L. 1998. HARKing: Hypothesizing after the results are known. *Personality and Social Psychology Review* 2(3). 196–217.

Kosmala, Loulou & Ludivine Crible. 2022. The dual status of filled pauses: Evidence from genre, proficiency and co-occurrence. *Language and Speech* 65(1). 216–239. DOI: 10.1177/00238309211010862.

Kosmala, Loulou & Aliyah Morgenstern. 2017. A preliminary study of hesitation phenomena in L1 and L2 productions: A multimodal approach. In *Disfluency in Spontaneous Speech 2017*.

Krüger, Martina. 2018. *Prosodic decoding and encoding of referential givenness in adults with autism spectrum disorders*. University of Cologne. (Doctoral dissertation).

Krüger, Martina, Francesco Cangemi, Kai Vogeley & Martine Grice. 2018. Prosodic marking of information status in adults with autism spectrum disorders. In *Proceedings of the 9th International Conference on Speech Prosody*, 182–186. Poznan, Poland.

Kügler, Frank, Bernadett Smolibocki, Denis Arnold, Stefan Baumann, Bettina Braun, Martine Grice, Stefanie Jannedy, Jan Michalsky, Oliver Niebuhr & Jörg Peters. 2015. DIMA: Annotation guidelines for German intonation. In *18. International Congress of Phonetic Sciences (ICPhS)*. Glasgow, UK.

Kuhl, Patricia K., Barbara T. Conboy, Sharon Coffey-Corina, Denise Padden, Maritza Rivera-Gaxiola & Tobey Nelson. 2008. Phonetic learning as a pathway to language: New data and native language magnet theory expanded (NLM-e). *Philosophical Transactions of the Royal Society B: Biological Sciences* 363(1493). 979–1000.

Kuiper, Lawrence. 1999. Parisian perceptions of regional French. *Handbook of perceptual dialectology* 1. 243–262.

Ladd, D. Robert. 2008. *Intonational phonology*. Cambridge, UK: Cambridge University Press.

Ladd, D. Robert, Kim EA Silverman, Frank Tolkmitt, Günther Bergmann & Klaus R. Scherer. 1985. Evidence for the independent function of intonation contour type, voice quality, and F0 range in signaling speaker affect. *The Journal of the Acoustical Society of America* 78(2). 435–444.

Ladd, D. Robert & J. M. B. Terken. 1995. Modelling intra-and inter-speaker pitch range variations. In *Proceedings of the XIIIth International Congress of Phonetic Sciences, ICPhS, Stockholm, Sweden*, 386–389.

Lai, Meng-Chuan, Michael V. Lombardo, Amber NV Ruigrok, Bhismadev Chakrabarti, Bonnie Auyeung, Peter Szatmari, Francesca Happé, Simon Baron-Cohen & MRC AIMS Consortium. 2017. Quantifying and exploring camouflaging in men and women with autism. *Autism* 21(6). 690–702.

Lake, Johanna K., Karin R. Humphreys & Shannon Cardy. 2011. Listener vs. Speaker-oriented aspects of speech: Studying the disfluencies of individuals with autism spectrum disorders. *Psychonomic Bulletin & Review* 18(1). 135–140.

Lee, Tzu-Lun, Ya-Fang He, Yun-Ju Huang, Shu-Chuan Tseng & Robert Eklund. 2004. Prolongation in spontaneous Mandarin. In *Interspeech ICSLP 2004, Jeju Island, South Korea*, vol. 3, 2181–2184.

Lehiste, Ilse. 1975. The phonetic structure of paragraphs. In A. Cohen & S. E.G. Noteboom (eds.), *Structure and process in speech perception*, 195–206. New York: Springer.

Lemoine, Nathan P. 2019. Moving beyond noninformative priors: Why and how to choose weakly informative priors in Bayesian analyses. *Oikos* 128(7). 912–928.

Leongómez, Juan David, Jakub Binter, Lydie Kubicová, Petra Stolařová, Kateřina Klapilová, Jan Havlíček & S. Craig Roberts. 2014. Vocal modulation during courtship increases proceptivity even in naive listeners. *Evolution and Human Behavior* 35(6). 489–496.

Levinson, Stephen C. 1983. *Pragmatics.* Cambridge, UK: Cambridge University Press.

Levinson, Stephen C. 2016. Turn-taking in human communication–origins and implications for language processing. *Trends in cognitive sciences* 20(1). 6–14.

Levinson, Stephen C. & Francisco Torreira. 2015. Timing in turn-taking and its implications for processing models of language. *Frontiers in psychology* 6. 731.

Levitan, Rivka, Stefan Benus, Agustin Gravano & Julia Hirschberg. 2015. Entrainment and turn-taking in human-human dialogue. In *AAAI Spring Symposia.*

Li, Han Z. 2006. Backchannel responses as misleading feedback in intercultural discourse. *Journal of Intercultural Communication Research* 35(2). 99–116.

Liberman, Alvin M., Franklin S. Cooper, Donal P. Shankweiler & Michael Studdert-Kennedy. 1967. Perception of the speech code. *Psychological Review* 74(6). 431–461. DOI: 10.1037/h0020279.

Linell, Per. 2004. *The written language bias in linguistics: Its nature, origins and transformations.* London, UK: Routledge.

Liu, Chang. 2013. Just noticeable difference of tone pitch contour change for English-and Chinese-native listeners. *The Journal of the Acoustical Society of America* 134(4). 3011–3020.

Liu, Huei-Mei, Patricia K. Kuhl & Feng-Ming Tsao. 2003. An association between mothers' speech clarity and infants' speech discrimination skills. *Developmental Science* 6(3). F1–F10.

Lord, Catherine, Eva Petkova, Vanessa Hus, Weijin Gan, Feihan Lu, Donna M. Martin, Opal Ousley, Lisa Guy, Raphael Bernier & Jennifer Gerdts. 2012. A multisite study of the clinical diagnosis of different autism spectrum disorders. *Archives of General Psychiatry* 69(3). 306–313.

Lord, Catherine, Susan Risi, Linda Lambrecht, Edwin H. Cook, Bennett L. Leventhal, Pamela C. DiLavore, Andrew Pickles & Michael Rutter. 2000. The Autism Diagnostic Observation Schedule—Generic: A Standard measure of social and communication deficits associated with the spectrum of autism. *Journal of Autism and Developmental Disorders* 30(3). 205–223.

Lucarini, Valeria, Francesco Cangemi, Benyamin Daniel Daniel, Jacopo Lucchese, Francesca Paraboschi, Chiara Cattani, Carlo Marchesi, Martine Grice, Kai Vogeley & Matteo Tonna. 2021. Conversational metrics, psychopathological dimensions and self-disturbances in patients with schizophrenia. *European Archives of Psychiatry and Clinical Neuroscience.* DOI: 10.1007/s00406-021-01329-w.

Lunsford, Rebecca, Peter A. Heeman, Lois Black & Jan van Santen. 2010. Autism and the use of fillers: Differences between ‘um’and ‘uh’. In *DiSS-LPSS Joint Workshop 2010.*

Matejka, Justin & George Fitzmaurice. 2017. Same stats, different graphs: Generating datasets with varied appearance and identical statistics through simulated annealing. In *Proceedings of the 2017 CHI Conference on Human Factors in Computing Systems*, 1290–1294.

McAleer, Phil, Alexander Todorov & Pascal Belin. 2014. How do you say ‘Hello’? Personality impressions from brief novel voices. *PLOS One* 9(3). e90779.

McCann, Joanne & Sue Peppé. 2003. Prosody in autism spectrum disorders: A critical review. *International Journal of Language & Communication Disorders* 38(4). 325–350.

McCleary, Leland & Tarcísio de Arantes Leite. 2013. Turn-taking in Brazilian sign language: Evidence from overlap. *Journal of Interactional Research in Communication Disorders* 4(1). 123.

McCracken, Chelsea. 2021. Autistic identity and language learning: Response to Kissine. *Language* 97(3). e211–e217. DOI: 10.1353/lan.2021.0038.

McElreath, Richard. 2020. *Statistical rethinking: A Bayesian course with examples in R and Stan (2nd edition).* London, UK: Chapman and Hall/CRC.

McGregor, Karla K. & Rex R. Hadden. 2020. Brief report:“Um” fillers distinguish children with and without ASD. *Journal of Autism and Developmental Disorders* 50(5). 1816–1821.

McShane, Blakeley B. & David Gal. 2017. Statistical significance and the dichotomization of evidence. *Journal of the American Statistical Association* 112(519). 885–895.
Megyesi, Beáta & Sofia Gustafson-Capková. 2002. Production and perception of pauses and their linguistic context in read and spontaneous speech in Swedish. In *Seventh International Conference on Spoken Language Processing*.
Mehu, Marc. 2011. Smiling and laughter in naturally occurring dyadic interactions: Relationship to conversation, body contacts, and displacement activities. *Human Ethology Bulletin* 26(1). 10–28.
Mennen, Ineke, Felix Schaeffler & Gerard Docherty. 2012. Cross-language differences in fundamental frequency range: A comparison of English and German. *The Journal of the Acoustical Society of America* 131(3). 2249–2260.
Mesch, Johanna. 2016. Manual backchannel responses in signers' conversations in Swedish Sign Language. *Language & Communication* 50. 22–41.
Milton, Damian. 2012. On the ontological status of autism: The 'double empathy problem'. *Disability & Society* 27(6). 883–887.
Milton, Damian. 2020. The double empathy problem. In *International Conference on "Neurodiversity: A Paradigm Shift In Higher Education & Employment" (2020)*.
Mitchell, Peter, Elizabeth Sheppard & Sarah Cassidy. 2021. Autism and the double empathy problem: Implications for development and mental health. *British Journal of Developmental Psychology* 39(1). 1–18. DOI: 10.1111/bjdp.12350.
Mohammadi, Gelareh, Antonio Origlia, Maurizio Filippone & Alessandro Vinciarelli. 2012. From speech to personality: Mapping voice quality and intonation into personality differences. In *Proceedings of the 20th ACM International Conference on Multimedia*, 789–792.
Mondada, Lorenza. 2019. Contemporary issues in conversation analysis: Embodiment and materiality, multimodality and multisensoriality in social interaction. *Journal of Pragmatics* 145. 47–62.
Morrison, Kerrianne E, Kilee M DeBrabander, Desiree R Jones, Daniel J Faso, Robert A Ackerman & Noah J Sasson. 2020. Outcomes of real-world social interaction for autistic adults paired with autistic compared to typically developing partners. *Autism* 24(5). 1067–1080. DOI: 10.1177/1362361319892701.
Murphy, Kevin R. & Herman Aguinis. 2019. HARKing: How badly can cherry-picking and question trolling produce bias in published results? *Journal of Business and Psychology* 34(1). 1–17.
Nadig, Aparna & Holly Shaw. 2012. Acoustic and perceptual measurement of expressive prosody in high-functioning autism: Increased pitch range and what

it means to listeners. *Journal of Autism and Developmental Disorders* 42(4). 499–511.

Nguyen, Vivian, Otto Versyp, Christopher Cox & Riccardo Fusaroli. 2022. A systematic review and Bayesian meta-analysis of the development of turn taking in adult–child vocal interactions. *Child Development* 93(4). 1181–1200. DOI: 10.1111/cdev.13754.

Nguyễn, Anh-Thư T. 2015. Acoustic correlates of listener-identified boundaries and prominences in spontaneous Vietnamese speech. *International Journal of Asian Language Processing* 25(2). 67–90.

Niebuhr, Oliver & Kerstin Fischer. 2019. Do not hesitate! – unless you do it shortly or nasally: How the phonetics of filled pauses determine their subjective frequency and perceived speaker performance. In *Interspeech 2019*, 544–548. ISCA. DOI: 10.21437/Interspeech.2019-1194.

Nolan, Francis. 2003. Intonational equivalence: An experimental evaluation of pitch scales. In *Proceedings of the 15th International Congress of Phonetic Sciences*, vol. 771. Barcelona,Spain.

Nolan, Francis. 2006. Intonation. In Bas Aarts & April McMahon (eds.), *The handbook of English linguistics*, 433–457. Oxford, UK: Blackwell.

O'Connell, Daniel C. & Sabine Kowal. 2004. The history of research on the filled pause as evidence of The Written Language Bias in Linguistics (Linell, 1982). *Journal of Psycholinguistic Research* 33(6). 459–474.

O'Shaughnessy, Douglas. 1992. Recognition of hesitations in spontaneous speech. In *IEEE International Conference on Acoustics, Speech, and Signal Processing*, vol. 1, 521–524. IEEE Computer Society.

Ochi, Keiko, Nobutaka Ono, Keiho Owada, Masaki Kojima, Miho Kuroda, Shigeki Sagayama & Hidenori Yamasue. 2019. Quantification of speech and synchrony in the conversation of adults with autism spectrum disorder. *PLOS ONE* 14(12). e0225377. DOI: 10.1371/journal.pone.0225377.

Ochs, Elinor, Tamar Kremer-Sadlik, Karen Gainer Sirota & Olga Solomon. 2004. Autism and the social world: An anthropological perspective. *Discourse Studies* 6(2). 147–183. DOI: 10.1177/1461445604041766.

Oertel, Catharine, Marcin Wlodarczak, Jens Edlund, Petra Wagner & Joakim Gustafson. 2012. Gaze patterns in turn-taking. In *Thirteenth Annual Conference of the International Speech Communication Association (ISCA)*.

Parish-Morris, Julia, Mark Y. Liberman, Christopher Cieri, John D. Herrington, Benjamin E. Yerys, Leila Bateman, Joseph Donaher, Emily Ferguson, Juhi Pandey & Robert T. Schultz. 2017. Linguistic camouflage in girls with autism spectrum disorder. *Molecular Autism* 8(1). 48. DOI: 10.1186/s13229-017-0164-6.

Patterson, David John. 2000. *A linguistic approach to pitch range modelling*. University of Edinburgh. (Doctoral dissertation).

Paul, Hermann. 1880. *Principien der Sprachgeschichte*, vol. 6. Tübingen: Niemeyer.

Paul, Rhea, Amy Augustyn, Ami Klin & Fred R. Volkmar. 2005. Perception and production of prosody by speakers with autism spectrum disorders. *Journal of Autism and Developmental Disorders* 35(2). 205–220.

Pietrowicz, Mary, Carla Agurto, Jonah Casebeer, Mark Hasegawa-Johnson, Karrie Karahalios & Guillermo Cecchi. 2019. Dimensional analysis of laughter in female conversational speech. In *ICASSP 2019-2019 IEEE International Conference on Acoustics, Speech and Signal Processing (ICASSP)*, 6600–6604. IEEE.

Pika, Simone, Ray Wilkinson, Kobin H. Kendrick & Sonja C. Vernes. 2018. Taking turns: Bridging the gap between human and animal communication. *Proceedings of the Royal Society B* 285(1880). 20180598.

Prechtel, Christine. 2023. *A cross-linguistic comparison of lexical stress strength and macro-rhythm strength*. University of California, Los Angeles. (Doctoral dissertation).

R Core Team. 2022. *R: A language and environment for statistical computing*. R Foundation for Statistical Computing. Vienna, Austria.

Rapin, Isabelle. 1991. Autistic children: Diagnosis and clinical features. *Pediatrics* 87(5). 751–760.

Ravignani, Andrea, Laura Verga & Michael D. Greenfield. 2019. Interactive rhythms across species: The evolutionary biology of animal chorusing and turn-taking. *Annals of the New York Academy of Sciences* 1453(1). 12–21. DOI: 10.1111/nyas.14230.

Reddy, Vasudevi, Emma Williams & Amy Vaughan. 2002. Sharing humour and laughter in autism and Down's syndrome. *British Journal of Psychology* 93(2). 219–242.

Rifai, Olivia M., Sue Fletcher-Watson, Lorena Jiménez-Sánchez & Catherine J. Crompton. 2022. Investigating markers of rapport in autistic and nonautistic interactions. *Autism in Adulthood* 4(1). 3–11. DOI: 10.1089/aut.2021.0017.

Roberts, Felicia & Alexander L. Francis. 2013. Identifying a temporal threshold of tolerance for silent gaps after requests. *The Journal of the Acoustical Society of America* 133(6). EL471–EL477.

Roettger, Timo B. 2019. Researcher degrees of freedom in phonetic research. *Laboratory Phonology: Journal of the Association for Laboratory Phonology* 10(1). DOI: 10.5334/labphon.147.

Roettger, Timo B., Bodo Winter & Harald Baayen. 2019. Emergent data analysis in phonetic sciences: Towards pluralism and reproducibility. *Journal of Phonetics* 73. 1–7.

RStudio Team. 2021. *RStudio: Integrated Development Environment for R*. RStudio, PBC. Boston, MA.

Ruch, Willibald & Paul Ekman. 2001. The expressive pattern of laughter. In A. Kaszniak (ed.), *Emotions, qualia, and consciousness*, 426–443. Tokyo, Japan: World Scientific Publishing.

Sacks, Harvey, Emanuel A. Schegloff & Gail Jefferson. 1974. A simplest systematics for the organization of turn taking for conversation. *Language* 50(4). 696–735.

Satzger, Wolfgang, Herbert Fessmann & Rolf R. Engel. 2002. Liefern HAWIE-R, WST und MWT-B vergleichbare IQ-Werte? *Zeitschrift für Differentielle und Diagnostische Psychologie* 23(2). 159–170.

Saubesty, Jorane & Marion Tellier. 2016. Multimodal analysis of hand gesture back-channel feedback. In *Gesture and Speech in Interaction 4*, 205–210.

Savino, Michelina. 2010. Intonational strategies for backchanneling in Italian Map Task dialogues. In *Third ISCA Workshop on Experimental Linguistics*.

Sawilowsky, Shlomo S. 2009. New effect size Rules of thumb. *Journal of Modern Applied Statistical Methods* 8(2). 26.

Sbranna, Simona, Francesco Cangemi & Martine Grice. 2021. Quantifying L2 interactional competence. *Language variation under contact conditions: Acquisitional contexts, languages, dialects and minorities in Italy and around the world – XVI AISV Conference Proceedings*.

Sbranna, Simona, Eduardo Möking, Simon Wehrle & Martine Grice. 2022. Backchannelling across languages: Rate, lexical choice and intonation in L1 Italian, L1 German and L2 German. *Proc. Speech Prosody 2022*. 734–738.

Sbranna, Simona, Simon Wehrle & Martine Grice. 2021. Developing L2 interactional competence: Turn-Taking across proficiency levels. In *Presentation at Phonetik und Phonologie im deutschsprachigen Raum, Frankfurt, Germany*.

Sbranna, Simona, Simon Wehrle & Martine Grice. 2023. The use of backchannels and other Very Short Utterances by Italian learners of German. In *Proceedings of XVIII AISV Conference "The Position of the Speaker in Interaction: Attitudes, Intentions, and Emotions in Verbal Communication"*. Naples, Italy.

Schegloff, Emanuel A. 1982. Discourse as an interactional achievement: Some uses of 'uh huh'and other things that come between sentences. In Deborah Tannen (ed.), *Analyzing discourse: Text and talk*, 71–93. Georgetown: Georgetown University Press.

Schegloff, Emanuel A. 1989. Reflections on language, development, and the interactional character of talk-in-interaction. In Marc H. Bornstein & Jerome S. Bruner (eds.), *Interaction in human development*, 139–153. Hillsdale, NJ: Lawrence Erlbaum.

Schegloff, Emanuel A. 2010. Some other "uh (m)" s. *Discourse Processes* 47(2). 130–174.
Schegloff, Emanuel A. 2020. Interaction: The infrastructure for social institutions, the natural ecological niche for language, and the arena in which culture is enacted. In Stephen J. Levinson & Nicholas J. Enfield (eds.), *Roots of human sociality*, 70–96. London, UK: Routledge.
Schegloff, Emanuel A., Gail Jefferson & Harvey Sacks. 1977. The preference for self-correction in the organization of repair in conversation. *Language* 53(2). 361–382.
Schettino, Loredana. 2019. Phonetic and functional features of lexicalized pauses in Italian. In *10th International Conference of Experimental Linguistics (ExLing 2019)*, 189–192. ExLing Society.
Schmidt, Karl-Heinz & Peter Metzler. 1992. *Wortschatztest (WST)*. Weinheim, Germany: Beltz.
Schnur, Tatiana T., Albert Costa & Alfonso Caramazza. 2006. Planning at the phonological level during sentence production. *Journal of Psycholinguistic Research* 35(2). 189–213.
Shannon, Claude E. 1948. A mathematical theory of communication. *The Bell System Technical Journal* 27(3). 379–423.
Sharda, Megha, T. Padma Subhadra, Sanchita Sahay, Chetan Nagaraja, Latika Singh, Ramesh Mishra, Amit Sen, Nidhi Singhal, Donna Erickson & Nandini C. Singh. 2010. Sounds of melody—Pitch patterns of speech in autism. *Neuroscience Letters* 478(1). 42–45.
Sheppard, Elizabeth, Dhanya Pillai, Genevieve Tze-Lynn Wong, Danielle Ropar & Peter Mitchell. 2016. How easy is it to read the minds of people with Autism Spectrum Disorder? *Journal of Autism and Developmental Disorders* 46(4). 1247–1254. DOI: 10.1007/s10803-015-2662-8.
Shriberg, Elizabeth. 2001. To 'errrr'is human: Ecology and acoustics of speech disfluencies. *Journal of the International Phonetic Association* 31(1). 153–169.
Shriberg, Elizabeth & Robin J. Lickley. 1993. Intonation of clause-internal filled pauses. *Phonetica* 50(3). 172–179.
Simmons, James Q. & Christiane Baltaxe. 1975. Language patterns of adolescent autistics. *Journal of Autism and Childhood Schizophrenia* 5(4). 333–351.
Smaldino, Paul E. & Richard McElreath. 2016. The natural selection of bad science. *Royal Society Open Science* 3(9). 160384.
Smith, Vicki L. & Herbert H. Clark. 1993. On the course of answering questions. *Journal of Memory and Language* 32(1). 25–38.
Sorace, Antonella. 2003. Near-nativeness. In C. J. Doughty & M. H. Long (eds.), *The handbook of second language acquisition*, 130–151. Oxford, UK: Blackwell.

Sørensen, Anna Josefine Munch, Michal Fereczkowski & Ewen N. MacDonald. 2019. Effects of noise and L2 on the timing of turn taking in conversation. In *Proceedings of the International Symposium on Auditory and Audiological Research*, vol. 7, 85–92.

Sóskuthy, Márton. 2021. Evaluating generalised additive mixed modelling strategies for dynamic speech analysis. *Journal of Phonetics* 84. 101017.

Spaniol, Malin, Alicia Janz, Simon Wehrle, Kai Vogeley & Martine Grice. 2023. Multimodal signalling: The interplay of oral and visual feedback in conversation. In *Proceedings of the 20th International Congress of Phonetic Sciences*. Prague, Czech Republic.

Sterling, Theodore D. 1959. Publication decisions and their possible effects on inferences drawn from tests of significance–or vice versa. *Journal of the American Statistical Association* 54(285). 30–34. DOI: 10.2307/2282137.

Sterponi, Laura, Kenton de Kirby & Jennifer Shankey. 2015. Rethinking language in autism. *Autism* 19(5). 517–526.

Stivers, Tanya, Nicholas J. Enfield, Penelope Brown, Christina Englert, Makoto Hayashi, Trine Heinemann, Gertie Hoymann, Federico Rossano, Jan Peter De Ruiter & Kyung-Eun Yoon. 2009. Universals and cultural variation in turn-taking in conversation. *Proceedings of the National Academy of Sciences* 106(26). 10587–10592.

Stocksmeier, Thorsten, Stefan Kopp & Dafydd Gibbon. 2007. Synthesis of prosodic attitudinal variants in German backchannel ja. In *Interspeech 2007*, 1290–1293. Antwerp, Belgium.

Suh, Joyce, Inge-Marie Eigsti, Letitia Naigles, Marianne Barton, Elizabeth Kelley & Deborah Fein. 2014. Narrative performance of optimal outcome children and adolescents with a history of an autism spectrum disorder (ASD). *Journal of Autism and Developmental Disorders* 44(7). 1681–1694.

Szatrowski, Polly. 2000. Relation between gaze, head nodding and aizuti 'back channel' at a Japanese company meeting. In *Annual Meeting of the Berkeley Linguistics Society*, vol. 26, 283–294.

Tager-Flusberg, Helen, Susan Calkins, Tina Nolin, Therese Baumberger, Marcia Anderson & Ann Chadwick-Dias. 1990. A longitudinal study of language acquisition in autistic and Down syndrome children. *Journal of Autism and Developmental Disorders* 20(1). 1–21.

Tager-Flusberg, Helen, Rhea Paul & Catherine Lord. 2005. Language and communication in autism. In F. Volkmar, R. Paul, A. Klin & D. J. Cohen (eds.), *Handbook of autism and pervasive developmental disorder*, 335–364. New York City, USA: John Wiley & Sons Inc.

Takahashi, Daniel Y., Alicia R. Fenley & Asif A. Ghazanfar. 2016. Early development of turn-taking with parents shapes vocal acoustics in infant marmoset monkeys. *Philosophical Transactions of the Royal Society B: Biological Sciences* 371(1693). 20150370.

Tepest, Ralf. 2021. The meaning of diagnosis for different designations in talking about autism. *Journal of Autism and Developmental Disorders* 51(2). 760–761. DOI: 10.1007/s10803-020-04584-3.

Thurber, Christopher & Helen Tager-Flusberg. 1993. Pauses in the narratives produced by autistic, mentally retarded, and normal children as an index of cognitive demand. *Journal of Autism and Developmental Disorders* 23(2). 309–322.

Torchiano, Marco. 2020. *Effsize: Efficient Effect Size Computation.* Manual. DOI: 10.5281/zenodo.1480624.

Torreira, Francisco & Sara Bögels. 2022. Vocal reaction times to speech offsets: Implications for processing models of conversational turn-taking. *Journal of Phonetics* 94. 101175. DOI: 10.1016/j.wocn.2022.101175.

Torreira, Francisco & Martine Grice. 2018. Melodic constructions in Spanish: Metrical structure determines the association properties of intonational tones. *Journal of the International Phonetic Association* 48(1). 9–32.

Tottie, Gunnel. 1991. Conversational style in British and American English: The case of backchannels. In Karin Aijmer & Bengt Altenberg (eds.), *English corpus linguistics*, 254–271. London, UK: Routledge.

Trouvain, Jürgen & Khiet P. Truong. 2017. Laughter. In Salvatore Attardo (ed.), *The Routledge handbook of language and humor*, 340–355. London, UK: Routledge.

Trouvain, Jürgen & Khiet P. Truong. 2012. Convergence of laughter in conversational speech: Effects of quantity, temporal alignment and imitation. In *International Symposium on Imitation and Convergence in Speech, Aix-en-Provence, France.*

Trouvain, Jürgen & Khiet P. Truong. 2013. Exploring sequences of speech and laughter activity using visualisations of conversations. In *Proceedings of the Workshop on Affective Social Speech Signals.*

Truong, Khiet P. & Jürgen Trouvain. 2012. On the acoustics of overlapping laughter in conversational speech. In *Thirteenth Annual Conference of the International Speech Communication Association.*

Tseng, Shu-Chuan. 2003. Taxonomy of spontaneous speech phenomena in Mandarin conversation. In *ISCA & IEEE Workshop on Spontaneous Speech Processing and Recognition.*

Tukey, John W. 1980. We need both exploratory and confirmatory. *The American Statistician* 34(1). 23–25.

Urbani, Martina. 2013. *The pitch range of Italians and Americans. A comparative study.* (Doctoral dissertation).
Vasishth, Shravan, Daniela Mertzen, Lena A. Jäger & Andrew Gelman. 2018. The statistical significance filter leads to overoptimistic expectations of replicability. *Journal of Memory and Language* 103. 151–175.
Vasishth, Shravan, Bruno Nicenboim, Mary E. Beckman, Fangfang Li & Eun Jong Kong. 2018. Bayesian data analysis in the phonetic sciences: A tutorial introduction. *Journal of Phonetics* 71. 147–161.
Vettin, Julia & Dietmar Todt. 2004. Laughter in conversation: Features of occurrence and acoustic structure. *Journal of Nonverbal Behavior* 28(2). 93–115.
Vivanti, Giacomo. 2020. Ask the editor: What is the most appropriate way to talk about individuals with a diagnosis of autism? *Journal of Autism and Developmental Disorders* 50(2). 691–693.
Vogel, David, Christine M. Falter-Wagner, Theresa Schoofs, Katharina Krämer, Christian Kupke & Kai Vogeley. 2019. Interrupted time experience in autism spectrum disorder: Empirical evidence from content analysis. *Journal of Autism and Developmental Disorders* 49(1). 22–33.
Vogel, David, Christine M. Falter-Wagner, Theresa Schoofs, Katharina Krämer, Christian Kupke & Kai Vogeley. 2020. Flow and structure of time experience–concept, empirical validation and implications for psychopathology. *Phenomenology and the Cognitive Sciences* 19(2). 235–258.
Ward, Nigel. 2000. Issues in the transcription of English conversational grunts. In *1st SIGdial Workshop on Discourse and Dialogue*, 29–35.
Ward, Nigel. 2006. Non-lexical conversational sounds in American English. *Pragmatics & Cognition* 14(1). 129–182.
Ward, Nigel. 2019. *Prosodic patterns in English conversation.* Cambridge, UK: Cambridge University Press.
Ward, Nigel & David DeVault. 2016. Challenges in building highly-interactive dialog systems. *AI Magazine* 37(4). 7–18.
Ward, Nigel, Rafael Escalante, Yaffa Al Bayyari & Thamar Solorio. 2007. Learning to show you're listening. *Computer Assisted Language Learning* 20(4). 385–407.
Ward, Nigel & Paola Gallardo. 2017. Non-native differences in prosodic-construction use. *Dialogue & Discourse* 8(1). 1–30.
Ward, Nigel & Wataru Tsukahara. 1999. A responsive dialog system. In Y. Wilks (ed.), *Machine conversations*, 169–174. Dordrecht, The Netherlands: Kluwer.
Ward, Nigel & Wataru Tsukahara. 2000. Prosodic features which cue back-channel responses in English and Japanese. *Journal of Pragmatics* 32(8). 1177–1207.

Warlaumont, Anne S., D. Kimbrough Oller, Rick Dale, Jeffrey A. Richards, Jill Gilkerson & Dongxin Xu. 2010. Vocal interaction dynamics of children with and without autism. In *Proceedings of the Annual Meeting of the Cognitive Science Society*, vol. 32.

Warlaumont, Anne S., Jeffrey A. Richards, Jill Gilkerson & D. Kimbrough Oller. 2014. A social feedback loop for speech development and its reduction in autism. *Psychological Science* 25(7). 1314–1324. DOI: 10.1177/0956797614531023.

Wehrle, Simon. 2022. *A brief tutorial for using Wiggliness and Spaciousness to measure intonation styles*. Retrievable online at https://osf.io/5e7fd. (14 December, 2022).

Wehrle, Simon, Francesco Cangemi, Harriet Hanekamp, Kai Vogeley & Martine Grice. 2020. Assessing the intonation style of speakers with Autism Spectrum Disorder. In *Proc. 10th International Conference on Speech Prosody 2020*, 809–813.

Wehrle, Simon, Francesco Cangemi, Alicia Janz, Kai Vogeley & Martine Grice. 2023. Turn-timing in conversations between autistic adults: Typical short-gap transitions are preferred, but not achieved instantly. *PLOS ONE* 18(4). e0284029. DOI: 10.1371/journal.pone.0284029.

Wehrle, Simon, Francesco Cangemi, Martina Krüger & Martine Grice. 2018. Somewhere over the spectrum: Between robotic and singsongy intonation. *Il parlato nel contesto naturale. Speech in the natural context* 4. 179–194. DOI: 10.17469/O2104AISV000010.

Wehrle, Simon, Francesco Cangemi, Kai Vogeley & Martine Grice. 2022. New evidence for melodic speech in Autism Spectrum Disorder. *Proc. Speech Prosody 2022*. 37–41.

Wehrle, Simon & Martine Grice. 2019. Function and prosodic form of backchannels in L1 and L2 German. In *Hanyang International Symposium on Phonetics and Cognitive Sciences of Language*. Seoul, South Korea.

Wehrle, Simon, Martine Grice & Kai Vogeley. 2023. Filled pauses produced by autistic adults differ in prosodic realisation, but not rate or lexical type. *Journal of Autism and Developmental Disorders*. DOI: 10.1007/s10803-023-06000-y.

Wehrle, Simon, Timo B. Roettger & Martine Grice. 2018. Exploring the dynamics of backchannel interpretation: The meandering mouse paradigm. In *ProsLang – Workshop on the Processing of Prosody across Languages and Varieties*. Wellington, New Zealand.

Wehrle, Simon & Christopher Sappok. 2023. Evaluating prosodic aspects of oral reading proficiency in schoolchildren: Effects of gender, genre and grade. In *Proceedings of the 20th International Congress of Phonetic Sciences*. Prague, Czech Republic.

Wehrle, Simon, Kai Vogeley & Martine Grice. 2023a. Backchannels in conversations between autistic adults are less frequent and less diverse prosodically and lexically. *Language and Cognition*. 1–26. DOI: 10.1017/langcog.2023.21.

Wehrle, Simon, Kai Vogeley & Martine Grice. 2023b. Characteristics and distribution of silent pauses in conversations between autistic and non-autistic dyads. In *Proceedings of the 20th International Congress of Phonetic Sciences*. Prague, Czech Republic.

Weilhammer, Karl & Susen Rabold. 2003. Durational aspects in turn taking. In *Proceedings of the 15th International Conference of Phonetic Sciences*. Barcelona, Spain.

Wesseling, Wieneke & Rob J. J.H. van Son. 2005. Early preparation of experimentally elicited minimal responses. In *6th SIGdial Workshop on Discourse and Dialogue*.

White, Sheida. 1989. Backchannels across cultures: A study of Americans and Japanese. *Language in Society* 18(1). 59–76.

Wickham, Hadley, Mara Averick, Jennifer Bryan, Winston Chang, Lucy D'Agostino McGowan, Romain François, Garrett Grolemund, Alex Hayes, Lionel Henry & Jim Hester. 2019. Welcome to the Tidyverse. *Journal of open source software* 4(43). 1686.

Wieling, Martijn, Jack Grieve, Gosse Bouma, Josef Fruehwald, John Coleman & Mark Liberman. 2016. Variation and change in the use of hesitation markers in Germanic languages. *Language Dynamics and Change* 6(2). 199–234.

Wilke, Claus O. 2020. *Cowplot: Streamlined Plot Theme and Plot Annotations for 'Ggplot2'*. Manual.

Wilke, Claus O. 2022. *Ggridges: Ridgeline Plots in 'Ggplot2'*. Manual.

Williams, Gemma L. 2021. Theory of autistic mind: A renewed relevance theoretic perspective on so-called autistic pragmatic 'impairment'. *Journal of Pragmatics* 180. 121–130. DOI: 10.1016/j.pragma.2021.04.032.

Williams, Gemma L., Tim Wharton & Caroline Jagoe. 2021. Mutual (mis)understanding: Reframing autistic pragmatic "impairments" using relevance theory. *Frontiers in Psychology* 12. DOI: 10.3389/fpsyg.2021.616664.

Winter, Bodo. 2014. Spoken language achieves robustness and evolvability by exploiting degeneracy and neutrality. *BioEssays* 36(10). 960–967. DOI: 10.1002/BIES.201400028.

Winter, Bodo & Paul-Christian Bürkner. 2021. Poisson regression for linguists: A tutorial introduction to modelling count data with brms. *Language and Linguistics Compass* 15(11). e12439.

Winter, Bodo & Martine Grice. 2021. Independence and generalizability in linguistics. *Linguistics* 59(5). 1251–1277.

Winter, Bodo & Andrew Wedel. 2016. The co-evolution of speech and the lexicon: The interaction of functional pressures, redundancy, and category variation. *Topics in Cognitive Science* 8(2). 503–513.

World Health Organization. 2022. *ICD-11: International statistical classification of diseases and related health problems.* World Health Organization.

Wozniak, Robert H., Nina B. Leezenbaum, Jessie B. Northrup, Kelsey L. West & Jana M. Iverson. 2017. The development of autism spectrum disorders: Variability and causal complexity. *Wiley Interdisciplinary Reviews: Cognitive Science* 8(1-2). e1426.

Xudong, Deng. 2008. The use of listener responses in Mandarin Chinese and Australian English conversations. *Pragmatics* 18(2). 303–328.

Yarkoni, Tal. 2022. The generalizability crisis. *Behavioral and Brain Sciences* 45. e1.

Yngve, Victor H. 1970. On getting a word in edgewise. In *Chicago Linguistics Society, 6th Meeting, 1970*, 567–578.

Yoshimura, Yuko, Koji Kawahara & Mitsuru Kikuchi. 2020. Turn-taking in children with Autism Spectrum Disorder: Discussion regarding ne and backchannel interjections. In *Japanese/Korean Linguistics Volume 26*, 3–11. Los Angeles: UCLA.

Young, Richard F. & Jina Lee. 2004. Identifying units in interaction: Reactive tokens in Korean and English conversations. *Journal of Sociolinguistics* 8(3). 380–407.

Yuan, Jiahong, Xiaoying Xu, Wei Lai & Mark Liberman. 2016. Pauses and pause fillers in Mandarin monologue speech: The effects of sex and proficiency. *Proceedings of Speech Prosody 2016.* 1167–1170.

Zellers, Margaret, David House & Simon Alexanderson. 2016. Prosody and hand gesture at turn boundaries in Swedish. *8th Speech Prosody 2016.* 831–835.

Zukauskas, Patricia Ribeiro, Francisco Baptista Assumpção Jr & Nava Silton. 2009. Temporality and Asperger's syndrome. *Journal of Phenomenological Psychology* 40(1). 85–106.

Name index